"There are secrets hiding in plain sight, so writes Dr. Lloyd Sederer in his new (10th!) book, which can make a real difference in the lives of people with mental and addictive disorders and their families. He is not only right; he reveals these secrets using stories, anecdotes, science, and history. This is a must and wonderful read for clinicians and for those affected by these all so common conditions."

Linda Rosenberg, *MSW, President and CEO, National Council for Behavioral Health*

"We've been honored to have Dr. Lloyd Sederer as a regular on my SiriusXM show to discuss his writings on mental health and addictions, as well as his film and book reviews. His expertise extends to every aspect of the human struggle with mental problems, from science to history, from popular culture to the drug war, as this Secrets book reveals. He is an uncommonly compassionate medical professional and public servant—and he's a terrific writer too."

John Fugelsang, *SiriusXM radio host*

IMPROVING MENTAL HEALTH
Four Secrets in Plain Sight

IMPROVING MENTAL HEALTH
Four Secrets in Plain Sight

Lloyd I. Sederer, M.D.

Medical Editor for Mental Health
of the Huffington Post and
Chief Medical Officer of the New York State Office
of Mental Health, New York, New York

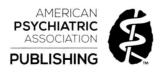

AMERICAN
PSYCHIATRIC
ASSOCIATION
PUBLISHING

Copyright © 2017 American Psychiatric Association
ALL RIGHTS RESERVED

Manufactured in the United States of America on acid-free paper
20 19 18 17 16   5 4 3 2 1
First Edition

American Psychiatric Association Publishing
1000 Wilson Boulevard
Arlington, VA 22209–3901
www.appi.org

Library of Congress Cataloging-in-Publication Data
Names: Sederer, Lloyd I., author. | American Psychiatric Association
  Publishing, publisher.
Title: Improving mental health : four secrets in plain sight / Lloyd I.
  Sederer.
Description: First edition. | Arlington, VA : American Psychiatric
  Association Publishing, [2017] | Includes bibliographical references.
Identifiers: LCCN 2016035449 (print) | LCCN 2016036324 (ebook) | ISBN
  9781615370825 (hc : alk. paper) | ISBN 9781615371204 (eb)
Subjects: | MESH: Mental Health | Mental Disorders--prevention & control |
  Stress, Psychological
Classification: LCC RC454 (print) | LCC RC454 (ebook) | NLM WM 101 | DDC
  616.89--dc23
LC record available at https://lccn.loc.gov/2016035449

British Library Cataloguing in Publication Data
A CIP record is available from the British Library.

For pilgrims and problem solvers around the world.

CONTENTS

FOREWORD

In the pages that follow, Lloyd I. Sederer, M.D., has distilled the lessons he has learned after more than 40 years of helping people with mental illness and addictions return to lives of love and contribution. As the Chief Medical Officer of the New York State Office of Mental Health, the nation's largest state mental health system, he has invaluable insights to share with the next generation of professionals and the patients and families they serve.

At the heart of his message is a fundamental recognition of the dignity and worth of each person—both practitioner and patient. As Dr. Sederer acknowledges, no one chooses to have a mental illness or addiction; we are all wired for human connection, to love and be accepted. Knowing the biological basis for these illnesses is only the first step in treating them, and the traditional medical response is only one leg of the stool. Any comprehensive treatment must include a strong psychosocial component.

Dr. Sederer effectively underscores that chronic stress—whether from childhood trauma, military service, or other sources—creates the conditions for brain illness. As a nation, we spend a great deal of time discussing the failures of our educational system, without understanding that adverse childhood experiences, or ACEs, such as living with an addicted or depressed parent or lacking basic necessities like food and housing, do serious damage to the developing brains of our country's children.

We must focus more attention on evidence-based interventions that can counter these early childhood experiences, promote brain fitness, support social and emotional development, and improve academic performance. Dr. Sederer is right to encourage mental health professionals to join with others to press for public policies that root out poverty, violence, discrimination, and other conditions that undermine the well-being of people at every stage of life.

Over the next decade, we will experience incredible breakthroughs in diagnosing and treating brain diseases. The future holds tremendous promise for learning more about genetic predispositions to behavioral health conditions, developing new, effective treatments with fewer side effects, and improving our ability to select the treatment that is most likely to work for a particular patient, among many innovations.

But the transformative changes our system needs will not simply depend on new tools and technologies. Rather, the biggest advances will come as a result of doing more of what we already know works. That is why the wisdom and guidance in *Improving Mental Health: Four Secrets in Plain Sight* are so important for professionals and patients who share Dr. Sederer's mission to achieve twenty-first-century mental health care for everyone who needs it.

Patrick J. Kennedy
June 2016

AUTHOR'S NOTE

The days were rainy, cool, and arduous. It was late October 2015, and my wife and I were on our annual hike working our way from central France to the west coast of northern Spain on the Santiago de Compostela Pilgrimage Trail. The trail is 1,600 kilometers, and we have walked, year after year a week at a time, about 1,000 kilometers so far.

I had just read Siddhartha Mukherjee's wonderful, short book *The Laws of Medicine: Field Notes from an Uncertain Science*. When you walk 8 hours a day, you have a lot of time to think. Inspired by this book about nature, medicine, and the three rather counterintuitive laws Mukherjee "discovered," I wondered what might be said of my field: mental health and addictions. What might make a difference for clinicians working with patients and families—and those directly affected as well—on their critical and heartbreaking issues?

Instead of laws, I reflected on four foundational truths, if you will, that I call secrets. They are insights from a long career, which are hidden in plain sight. I imagined a book of patient stories, historical incidents and notable people, books and movies, and research findings to reveal and illuminate each of the four proposed secrets. I wanted to convey to practicing psychiatrists, general medical and pediatric doc-

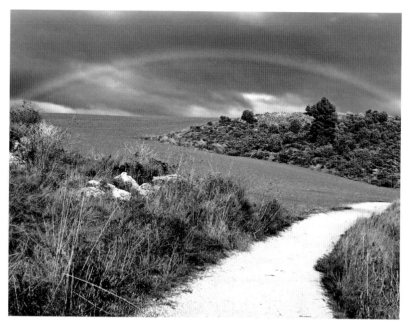

The Camino, West of Pamplona, Spain.

tors, psychologists, social workers, counselors, nurses, and trainees in all of these disciplines what they could do more of in everyday practice. I wanted to speak to people with mental disorders and their loved ones about what they too can do to make an immediate difference in their lives. I jotted some notes as I walked and talked about them with my wife, one of the best writers I know. In a couple of days, I had the design for this book and its principal themes.

I want to recognize, as well, not just the inspiration of Dr. Mukherjee's book but the encouragement he offered me when I wrote to him about the book that I had in mind. That was more than I needed to get started.

The "secrets" that I believe are there for all of us to see and apply are as follows: 1) behavior serves a purpose; 2) the power of attachment; 3) as a rule, less is more; and 4) chronic stress is the enemy.

I also wanted to write a short book, not hundreds of pages but a fraction of that. I was reminded of aphorisms about how easy it can be to write a long speech or article and how hard composing a short one can be. As a writer and teacher, I thought about the competing demands upon the time and attention of those for whom I write. I aim to communicate with them in ways that are concise, clear, and—I hope—engaging as well.

I remain optimistic for further and important scientific advances in my field, despite what has been their languorous pace. But I see daily that we already know so much about what works. Practitioners in my field can do so much more by reducing the gap between what we know and what we do. The secrets in this book reveal a way to close the science-to-practice gap. They are meant to illustrate opportunities in plain sight by which clinicians can help patients and families and through which individuals can help themselves take the kinds of actions that will enable them to have better, richer lives—right now.

INTRODUCTION

If cancer is the emperor of all maladies, with all due respect to those conditions and their modern day archivist Dr. Siddhartha Mukherjee, then mental illness is their Zeus. Mental (and addictive) disorders are ubiquitous, psychically devastating, responsible for enormous family and social burdens as well as economic costs, and too often defy cure. Mental illness is, unfortunately, a far greater affliction than cancer in terms of its consequences.

This is not merely a matter of pride of place for the conditions that so markedly cast a shadow over the human and medical landscape. It is also a matter of how limited our successes have been, over centuries, to reduce the pain, suffering, and prevalence of the conditions that so greatly impact our lives. The scorecards—the results—for those efforts must be improved.

As a young doctor and psychiatrist over 40 years ago, I was awed by the endless capabilities of the human brain's billions of cells and trillions of connections and by the mind's depths and reaches. I was intrigued by the illnesses that plague the mind—whose history is even more ancient and grim than that of cancer. Since then, as a practicing psychiatrist and clinical administrator, I have treated and supervised the care of tens of thousands of patients. Today, as a public health doctor, I develop and implement policies and programs that can reach hundreds of thousands of people each year. I remain hopeful for scientific advances despite what has been their languorous pace, yet I am saddened by recognizing that we already know so much about what works but are very far from realizing the benefits of our knowledge.

I knew an accomplished attorney, a man in his mid-50s, who had worked for my parents years ago. After their deaths, I tried to contact him about some legal matters that he had consulted upon. When I called his office, I was transferred to the managing partner of his firm, who told me in a whispered voice that he had died. When I inquired further, and the partner learned that I was a psychiatrist, out poured the tragic story of his suicide. He had become depressed, resisted treatment, and was anxiously avoided by his colleagues and friends, who did not know what to say or do. He became unable to work. His depression deepened, and with access to a deadly means of killing himself, he proceeded to do so.

His loss—consider also Robin Williams and too many others—was likely avoidable. Treatment for depression works. Prevention of suicide is possible by detecting and treating the underlying mental (and/or addictive) disorder and by establishing safety plans, which include enhancing the emotionally protective aspects of a person's life and reducing access to deadly implements, especially guns. Families can learn how to help their loved ones, as can friends and colleagues. But this happens far too infrequently. Fewer than one in five people with depression are diagnosed and receive what has been termed "minimally effective care" (in terms of therapy and/or medications). More than 42,000 people annually die by their own hands in the United States; the numbers continue to rise every year. Of the 10 most preventable causes of death, only suicide rates continue to increase.

I believe that the greatest gains in the next 10 years for people with mental and addictive disorders, and their families, will come from better executing what we now know. Habit often stands in the way of carrying this out. We must recognize and be willing to discard the habits of ineffective practices and dated ideas that obscure the secrets that I identify. When we effectively reach more people with prevention, treatments, and health maintenance strategies that work, we will greatly improve the lives of millions of people. This has been called closing the science-to-practice gap: translating into everyday practice the clinical and program research results proven to be effective. We will know when we have closed that gap when someone with an illness can readily and reliably access proven treatments at any mental health or medical office, clinic, or hospital. We will see great leaps forward in public mental health in the years ahead when we find ways to do more of what we already know works.

Part and parcel of closing the science-to-practice gap is a set of *fundamental ways by which everyday mental health practices can be improved. In this book we will consider* **four secrets** *of mental health care* that can make that difference now. I want to convey them to mental health practitioners, clinical leaders, and graduate students. I want to convey them to those individuals and families affected by mental disorders who want to amplify their voices in clinical encounters by knowing what counts in their treatment and in their lives.

John Clement, a 17-year-old boy whose early adolescence glowed with sports and school success, has hardly left his room, spoken with friends or family, or showered in months. He stays up all night and screams chilling cries at unpredictable moments to unknown listeners. His parents and older sister know something is terribly wrong but cannot understand his behaviors—why he would act this way. They exhort him to go to school, come to dinner, put on clean clothes.

Introduction

The more they push, the more he digs in: every action has an equal and opposite reaction. They are embarrassed to ask for help, don't know where to turn or whom to trust with what is breaking their hearts.

John's behaviors make sense once we understand what is going on in his mind. But he is shut tighter than a drum. John is not going to explain why he behaves bizarrely; in fact, that's not how he sees it. It is we who don't understand, he thinks. The **first secret** we need to appreciate is that **behavior serves a purpose**. John is acting as he does because his avoidance, his fearful behaviors, his screams are the ways that he is trying to manage how he is feeling and thinking. Not very effective, but the best way he has, so far. His family and many others have yet to comprehend what purposes his behaviors serve. When they do, the dissension a family experiences can lessen and lead to discussion—to figuring out how to best respond to a person experiencing psychic distress and disordered thoughts. Looking for meaning and communicating purpose in behaviors is a too often overlooked aspect of mental health care and a lost opportunity for patients and their families.

A hundred years ago, in Europe and then throughout the Western world, a Viennese neurologist named Sigmund Freud was publishing riveting stories in the form of tales from the couch. His narratives made the case for a theory of the mind in which our drives, particularly sex (eros) and aggression, commanded our actions as well as those, he later hypothesized, of civilization itself. He was teaching us about human motivation and its vicissitudes. However, this aspect of Freud's work would, a few decades later, be overturned by French and American developmental psychologists whose studies illuminated the even greater power of our relationships, our "fierce attachments," as the writer Vivian Gornick called them. Time has only more firmly rooted this awareness of the power of **attachment as a human need and drive** into the study of human relations. That is the **second secret**.

This second secret is actionable in clinical care: it needs to be harnessed if we are to change painful and problem behaviors. Relationships are the royal road to remedying human suffering, indeed a highway to changing civilization as well. Mothers will die for their child, and soldiers will die for a combat buddy. Because survival is our most basic and universal motivation, overcoming that drive for the welfare of another person makes the case for the power of attachment. In Chapter 2, "The Power of Attachment," we will look at other examples as well.

The **third secret** of mental health practice should hardly be a secret. But so often it is. **As a rule, less is more,** which means that when we can make do with less, then, in fact, we often have done more. Mental health treatments, biological and psychosocial, as well as many medical treatments, have been aggressive in their therapeutic approaches. High doses of drugs for schizophrenia or leukemia illustrate doctors trying to wipe out illnesses—wanting to do as much as possible, when less not only might do as well (or better) and would produce reduced suffering and far greater tolerance of the treatment by those subject to it. I recall working at a Harvard teaching hospital when the ethos of the treatment for psychosis was "hit them with industrial strength doses of antipsychotics." A similar approach, for many years, characterized mastectomies. Doing more in terms of frequency of visits and/or psychic confrontation has been, as well, an approach for some types of individual and group psychotherapy. These were not bad doctors or clinicians at work. However, they followed a school of thought that posited if a little works, then more will work better. Knowing the third secret will open our eyes to better and more successful care.

Maria Anton, age 13, is pregnant and failing in school. She is obese, smokes, and is showing metabolic evidence of insulin insensitivity, a precursor to diabetes. She has been diagnosed as having depression and has already had an acetaminophen (Tylenol) overdose after a disappointment with her boyfriend. She was raised in foster care from age five after she was abused by her stepfather and her mother was unable to care for her because of a crack cocaine addiction. (Sederer 2016, p. 235)

Children are at exponentially greater risk of general medical and mental illnesses by adolescence or young adulthood if they are exposed to the stressors of physical, emotional, and sexual abuse; neglect; parental separation or divorce; mental illness or substance use disorder; incarceration of a household member; or domestic violence. These are called adverse childhood experiences (ACEs), and the presence of each one compounds the others in terms of increasing risk. A robust body of evidence demonstrates the grave lifelong blows that adverse childhood experiences deliver.

The **fourth secret** is that **chronic stress is the enemy**. ACEs are but one way that chronic mental and physical stresses (which are inseparable) are induced. Recent evidence on posttraumatic stress disorder also points strongly to the body's stress response as the underlying mechanism in the pathogenesis of this "page 1" illness. Depression, diabetes, hypertension, and heart disease are not exceptions to this stress-disease relationship. Chronic stress can be reduced and managed—and its damage prevented or diminished. The fourth secret is eminently actionable, as well.

These are secrets hiding in plain sight. Each one, unveiled and freed from the constraints of ineffective habits and behaviors, can change lives. Together, when revealed and acted upon, they can change the world. That's why I wrote this book.

Reference

Sederer LS: The social determinants of mental health. Psychiatr Serv 67(2):234–235, 2016 26522677

CHAPTER 1

BEHAVIOR SERVES A PURPOSE

We don't see things as they are,
we see things as we are.

Anaïs Nin

One doesn't discover new lands
without consenting to lose sight
of the shore for a very long time.

André Gide

I believe behavior serves a purpose. But often, particularly for people with mental and addiction disorders, that purpose is not at all clear or straightforward. Frequently, the person affected may not know what is driving his or her behavior. However, it is possible to discern, with careful, nonjudgmental listening and thoughtful questioning, what purpose is served by a person acting or refusing to act.

Irene Maxwell was a single mom in her early 50s with two teenage daughters. She worked as an office manager for a small company and oversaw a well-run home, believing this was essential to keeping kids from the many ways they can stray and thereby not succeed at school and life. However, after a long bout of the winter flu and the onset of menopausal symptoms that awakened her at night in a sweat, she began to miss a day here and there from work. Dinner was not always on the table at 7:00 P.M. as was her custom. She took fewer pains with her appearance, began to be late and forgetful, and worried a lot. Then one day she could not bring herself to go to work—not just for a day but for the foreseeable future.

Her children implored her to get off the couch, to do something other than lie around and fret. Her sister and her best friend warned Ms. Maxwell that she could lose her job unless she returned to work. But she knew all that. In fact, knowing that she needed to function and fearing unemployment added to her paralysis, it didn't help to rally her. She became even more immobilized and felt hopeless.

At first, Ms. Maxwell had been able to force herself to go to work. But she discovered that once there, she could not concentrate; she sat at her desk pushing papers around and not getting anything done. She couldn't pay attention at meetings and began to miss deadlines. She

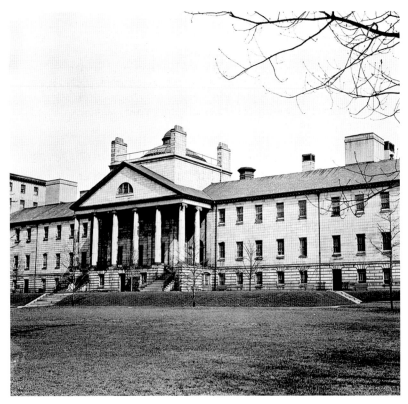

Original Massachusetts General Hospital.

was mortified. She thought if her boss and coworkers saw more of her failings, she would surely lose her job. She, like so many of us, "managed" her shame and anxiety about her poor performance by the most common technique known to humankind, namely, avoidance. Not only would she be spared what felt like the huge burden of getting up on time, showering, and preparing for and traveling to work, she also could escape the disgrace of not living up to her own standards of hard work responsibly done.

Ms. Maxwell was staying home not because she was lazy or bad. Her behavior served the purpose of sparing her further shame and failure. Of course, this was a short-lived and ineffective solution to her problems, which she kept to herself, but she did not know (then) any better way of coping, and she did not believe anything could help.

Human behavior has long been considered psychologically overdetermined, a term dating back to early psychoanalysis. When any of us acts, it is generally the result of a variety of motives and psychological forces. When I provide examples here, I mean to be illustrative not exhaustive in describing what may be an array of forces at work.

It is essential for clinicians and loved ones to appreciate what purpose or purposes are served when a person with a mental illness engages in behaviors that seem to defy reason. Doing so enables us all to eschew blaming and to provide the empathy and support that can begin to help the person affected find better, less compromised solutions.

Hateful Patients

"Admitted or not, the fact remains that a few patients kindle aversion, fear, despair or even outright malice in their doctors," wrote Dr. James Groves in the *New England Journal of Medicine* in 1978 (Groves 1978, p. 883). His paper was called "Taking Care of the Hateful Patient." Jim was working as a psychiatrist on the medical-surgical wards of Massachusetts General Hospital, where I came to know him because I was directing the hospital's inpatient psychiatric unit. His paper was sensational because it was so candid in its admission of what doctors feel and seldom reveal. It was also very helpful to doctors, as well as to patients and their families.

Dr. Groves described those patients he observed who were the most hated by his medical colleagues. He denoted four patient categories: the dependent clingers; the entitled demanders; the manipulative help-rejecters; and the self-destructive deniers. He wanted to help doctors stick with difficult patients, to escape a sense of helplessness that can befall practitioners when trying to care for those patients who seem to regularly defeat their doctors—as well as nurses and other professionals (not to mention the patients themselves). His careful depictions of these varied "hateful" patients revealed one thing that they had in common: their behaviors served a purpose.

Patients characterized as dependent clingers can feel inescapable to their caregivers. They seem to be always there, waiting to ruin the doctor's day, but their purpose is to be seen and responded to. Oblivious to the effect of their relentless cries for attention, they can exhaust and alienate many a physician. Whether these patients have a frivolous or grave problem is not relevant, although, of course, the patients with the more serious conditions have far more to lose. But their desire—to be cared for, to draw succor from a seemingly inexhaustible medical well—drives them and defeats their efforts to obtain the very nurture they so desperately seek.

Entitled demanders test the most dedicated caregivers. Their hostile, devaluing methods evoke revulsion and intense aversion. What purpose can that serve? Groves remarks that they are in "terror of abandonment," which is buried beneath their offensive sense of superiority.

The more they demand, the less likely they will be successful, but this escapes their reasoning and capacity to act in ways that might better serve their self-interest. Groves offers a clinical strategy that "goes with" the entitlement rather than confronting it. He suggests channeling the demands of these individuals toward more reasonable expectations of "first-rate medical care," a type of linguistic jujitsu. When effective, patients are not abandoned or avoided and the delivery of good care stands a chance. That's good for patients, not just doctors.

"Crocks" has long been a term among medical professionals, disparaging as it may be. However, using the term is one way doctors, nurses, and others try to cope with those patients who reject help, who seem to be determined to defeat those trying to care for them. These patients can seem manipulative too (hence the term manipulative help-rejecters) because they are so profoundly dependent that they will do anything, or do nothing, in order to come back—again and again—seeking more, which is their objective. In Yiddish, there is an expression, *gornish helfin*, which means nothing will help. That's the song of the help-rejecters. Seeing the doctor can be far more important than getting better; it is critical to understand this as the purpose driving the patients' behavior. They live in a psychic world diametrically opposed to their caregivers, who want to see improvements, and this makes them especially trying. But their purpose becomes more clear—and thus more helpful to patients—when we clinicians are able to look past our own reactions, when we don't try to explain the behavior to these patients but, instead, practice humility—when we say that we can only do our best and the rest is in their hands.

Finally, Groves' nosology gives us the self-destructive deniers. These are patients, for example, who continue to abuse alcohol despite having severe liver failure and swollen esophageal veins that are ready to pop. These patients are managing a fear of ever getting better, of ever living a life with others, by aggressively rejecting any such possibility. Yet again, what might seem inexplicable and hateful serves a purpose; it's just a different purpose from what the patient-doctor relationship ostensibly calls for. These are people willing to die before they will risk trying to live. Some doctors feel so angry with these self-destructive deniers that they can't help but wish the patients would, in fact, just die. What cannot work with these patients is a contest to win them over; only *they* can choose to join the living, or try to. Motivational interviewing techniques (techniques not in wide use when Groves wrote his article), first used with people with addiction problems and now also popular in primary care, are effective ways to keep the doctor from "losing it" with these patients. Motivational interviewing is a way to stand a chance with them, to move patients from "no way" to "maybe" when it comes to their self-care. Motivational interviewing is based on the notion that behavior is purposeful: clinicians start by believing that how a person is acting must be doing *something* for them. By not allowing patients to dismiss that premise and derail the clinical inquiry, with time and a nonjudgmental stance, the "why" of patients' behavior can emerge. That is the moment for clinicians to go further and ask, "How's that working for you?" That is the moment to tip the psychological seesaw from the painful present to a different and more successful future.

As a psychiatrist spending his days and nights on the medical-surgical wards (and outpatient clinics) of a general hospital, Dr. Groves was able to identify those exasperating patients who made the work of his colleagues the most difficult. It was not just the hard work of caring for patients, he remarked, that could exhaust caregivers; it was the additional burden of their hateful, aversive feelings that could make the clinician's job unbearable and unsustainable. He was writing to look after his fellow caregivers so they, in turn, could do the work they wanted to do, namely, take care of the patient, even when he or she is hateful. And Jim was teaching us all that behavior serves a purpose that can be discerned and dealt with in ways that better serve the patient and the doctor as well.

The Myth of Mental Illness

I was a medical student in 1968 on rotation in psychiatry when I attended a seminar by Dr. Thomas Szasz. I was astounded by his erudition and mental alacrity. A forced refugee, he fled the Nazis in 1938. He excelled in college, medical school, and psychiatric training in the United States and served in the U.S. Navy, despite having arrived here not speaking a word of English. In 1961, he published one of the most groundbreaking books in my field and possibly in the social and political sciences: *The Myth of Mental Illness* (Szasz 1961)

Many regard Szasz as antipsychiatry, and, indeed, he was one of my field's most vocal critics. However, seeing him as antipsychiatry reveals a casual reader's view of his work—or perhaps a wish to promote a perspective of psychiatry as dangerous to your liberty, if not your health. His contributions were far greater than that. My education with Thomas Szasz continued through my residency and then as a colleague until he died, in 2012, at the age of 92. He was one who surely understood that behavior serves a purpose.

In *The Myth of Mental Illness*, Szasz, a classically trained psychoanalyst, illustrates how behaviors that are often seen as mental illnesses can be understood in ways that eluded comprehension at the time psychiatry was born in the early twentieth century. One case that Szasz explores in the book is that of a 24-year-old woman, the third daughter in a prosperous family, Fräulein Elizabeth Von R, who had consulted the then-little-known Viennese neurologist, Sigmund Freud, in 1892 for a hysterical conversion (which was not uncommon at that time).

Conversion symptoms include blindness, paralysis, seizures, and pain; they appear in the absence of any underlying neurological pathology. The Fräulein had leg pain accompanied by difficulty walking. Her skin and leg muscles were *hyperalgesic*, highly tender and painful when touched. Freud observed, however, that her reaction to pain when elicited, say, by touch, appeared to be one more of pleasure than pain. He then theorized from his psychoanalysis of her that her conversion symptoms were erotic in nature and disguised her hidden love for her brother-in-law.

Dr. Szasz, too, posited that the Fräulein indeed had a mental problem, but he regarded it as one of *communication*. She, he claims, was changing (converting if you will) a personal problem to a body problem through the use of *protolanguage*: a lower or earlier form of language than words. Protolanguages are the lexicon of less sophisticated people or, as in the case of this young woman, of those who are powerless to express themselves directly. Szasz argues that hysterical symptoms transmit a message, through the body, that serves multiple functions. The physical symptoms can make what seems a devil of a problem more manageable or at least more discrete (and perhaps discreet as well!).

According to the work, which Szasz summarizes, of Hans Reichenbach, a Jewish activist and academic from Berlin who also fled Hitler and became an American philosopher of science and logic, the three functions that a protolanguage can serve are *informative*, *affective*, and *promotive*. The informative function tells the listener (or the observer) "I am sick," "I am disabled," "I need help." Simultaneously, the body message also evokes feelings (affects) in whomever receives the message, including family, friends, and doctors. Commonly, we feel sorry for the person afflicted, and we are not prone to judge them. The final function, fostered by the other two, encourages the observer to act, to do something on behalf of the sufferer: the observer is moved to take care of or to treat the person who is in pain or disabled, to absolve them of any blame, or merely to leave them alone.

This potent communication triplet is a remarkable display of how a behavior, psychologically produced, serves many purposes. The unconscious intelligence and purposefulness of protolanguage is quite awesome, for we witness how a mind foreclosed from one form of communication will find another. Such communications, moreover, are protective; the person conveying their hidden message is not very open to attack or even to disappointment because, after all, they have not manifestly asked for anything!

The coup de grâce of protolanguage communications is that these communications manage, however indirectly and with a poor chance of solving any actual dilemma, to sustain the relationship with the needed other. Here we see how what later psychologists and psychoanalysts called the *object relationship*, our fundamental need for attachment (discussed in detail in Chapter 2, "The Power of Attachment"), is beautifully served. No human tie is broken with protolanguage; for at least a while, the relationship is maintained despite what could threaten to sever it, namely, the interpersonal problem that spawned it in the first place.

Szasz was in this writing, and throughout his long and prolific career, deeply concerned about inequity in human relations, all the more so when one person or group is dominated or oppressed by another, others, or the government that is meant to serve them. Conversion reactions thus portrayed—in this case and for the many women who experienced them in the nineteenth and into the twentieth century—how women were subjugated and unable to express themselves, except through their bodies. Dr. Szasz, I think, was among the early feminists in his writings.

Neurasthenia is a psychological disorder characterized by fatigability, lack of motivation, feelings of inadequacy, and psychosomatic symptoms. This condition, described by Dr. Silas Weir Mitchell, a prominent Philadelphia physician in the late 1800s who prescribed the "rest cure" for women, is another example of how able but socially handcuffed women were diagnosed and dismissed.

These reactions and responses do not, however, fix the problem. In conversions, neurasthenia, some pain syndromes, and other psychological means by which those of lesser status express themselves, the underlying problem—the inequity of the relationship, the interpersonal dominance that oppresses and gags proper expression—is not remedied. Good psychiatric treatment, thus, starts with the premise and the psychotherapeutic practice that a better language is needed to achieve a more just relationship. The freedom to express ourselves and the freedom to pursue what is fair are among the cornerstones of good mental health treatment. This is made possible when a clinician, as well as the patient and family members, appreciates how behavior serves a purpose.

Psychotic Conditions and Eating Disorders

Two conditions particularly puzzle and thwart clinicians as well as families. The first condition is a **psychotic illness**, particularly schizophrenia, schizoaffective disorder, or excited bipolar states, in which everyday reality is eclipsed by delusional thinking, in which behaviors become bizarre, seemingly inexplicable, and even dangerous to the person who is ill and, on occasion, to family members and even strangers. The other condition, which tends to occur in young people, teenage girls and boys, is the eating disorder called **anorexia nervosa**. How can these often smart youth pursue a relentless starvation campaign? How can they not yield to what we know to be the urgent pangs of hunger and the obvious wasting that their body broadcasts to any onlooker? The behaviors that derive from both of these illnesses serve a purpose, although sweet reason usually does not readily recognize what that may be. Let's look at each of these in turn, beginning with psychosis.

Psychosis

Psychotic behavior often confounds our understanding. How can a teenage girl, a good student and friend, avoid her friends, stop taking care of herself, and refuse to go to school? How can a twenty-something son board himself up in his room, chain smoke cigarettes, and yell piercing screams at night? How can (as does happen and chills us all) a mother take the life of her young child or children?

Two interlocking mental processes underlie these behaviors: one drives the behaviors and the other renders them so difficult to alter. The first process, often described as a symptom, is characterized by *delusions*, fixed ideas that a person develops, which fly in the face of the reality that others are fortunate to be able to discern. The second is distinguished by an *inability* of a person to appreciate that he or she is indeed acting under the sway of a delusion, including one that can destroy his or her life and threaten the well-being of others.

Ruth Brooke was 45 when I saw her for evaluation when practicing in Massachusetts years ago. She was an accomplished professional who had suffered from **bipolar disorde**r since her mid-20s. Her condition was unstable; treatment was not containing her mood swings, which impaired her ability to work and which were highly disruptive at home and to her marriage. Her husband attended the evaluation and offered to be helpful in any ways he could. I reviewed options for a different treatment approach with them and arranged to see her again in a week. But a few days later, I received a call from her husband and sister saying she had become very ill: she was destroying property in her home and menacing her family. I prepared commitment papers (thinking I would need them) and by phone arranged for the police in her town outside Boston to meet me at her home, where family members would be waiting.

I arrived about 9:00 at night. Her husband and sister were there, as were the local police. We huddled in the lights of parked cars. I knocked at the door to enter, but Mrs. Brooke was screaming and threatened me. She said nothing was the matter with her, that she had work to do, and that her husband—and now I—was getting in the way of her discovering a solution to a common and deadly form of cancer. I called for an ambulance and arranged for her admission to a psychiatric hospital in the area. When the police went to the door, she quieted considerably and went peaceably, but in restraints, with the ambulance personnel and was taken to a psychiatric hospital, where she was involuntarily admitted. A few days later, her husband called me to thank me for my intervention and to say that his wife was doing better. He added that she never wanted to see me again.

The manic delusion Ruth Brooke was under was grandiose in nature. She believed that she, with no research background or experience in a laboratory, was going to crack the code and cure cancer. Her long-standing disposition to be a helper and a comforter to others had become amplified beyond reason as a result of her mania. Her illness had rapidly escalated; she was in a sleepless and agitated state; and her family's efforts to talk with her evoked aggressive responses. To her mind, however, she had cause to be explosive because those around her could not appreciate the medical gift she was about to give countless families—not to mention the struggling scientists who could not match her brilliance. This helps to explain her aggressive determination, to the point of violence even, to act on her delusions. Initially, it would take a biological intervention, antimanic and antipsychotic medication, to return her to her previously high-functioning and pacific self. However, her profound inability to know she had relapsed into mania required what is always the least desired intervention, namely, taking away her liberty and treating her, for what was a matter of days, until reason could once again prevail. Her behavior in a manic state was meant to serve the delusional belief she had developed and to pursue humanitarian aims, however misguided. It all made sense to her; it was her mission. Only treatment could alter the aberrant but purposeful mind-set that preoccupied her.

Psychotic depression also can produce behaviors that boggle the mind. One of the most chilling examples in this century involved Andrea Yates, a Texas mother of five children, who confessed, in 2001, to drowning them in her bathtub. She was suffering from postpartum psychosis, likely a schizoaffective disorder, according to the defense psychiatrist involved in her second court trial.

In 2001, during an episode of postpartum psychosis (called that because of its temporal relationship to the time after a woman gives birth), Andrea Yates felt the presence of Satan. He directed her to drown her children in the bathtub of her Houston, Texas, home in order to save them from burning in the fires of hell. If she killed them, she believed, they would go to heaven—a place of peace and comfort for them.

Yates had been a good mother, a nurse. She homeschooled her five children, including teaching them Bible lessons. The act of taking their lives, as horrific as that was, makes some sense if we consider that a "good" mother would try to save her children from an eternity of pain and hellfire. We can speculate that her illness left her profoundly unable to care for her children, and that unbearable state might have driven her to relieve them of their misery, as her hallucinations demanded. At her first trial, Andrea Yates was found "not insane" (the term used in court proceedings) and guilty of capital murder; she was

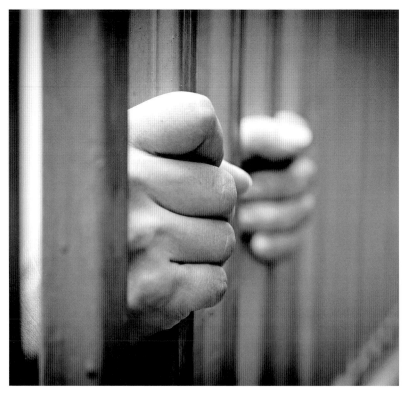

U.S . prison.

then sentenced to life in prison. However, because of erroneous testimony by an expert witness, the conviction was appealed and reversed. In 2006, after 5 years in prison, she was found "not guilty by reason of insanity" and remanded to a forensic psychiatric facility, where she remains to this day.

Yates suffered from severe, intermittent depression but had difficulty taking the medications that helped her mood and controlled her psychotic thinking, in part because she stopped the medications during her repeated pregnancies. After the birth of her fifth child, Mary, in 2000 and the death of her father in 2001, she became psychotic and deeply obsessed with religion. She was paranoid, saw cameras in the ceiling, and underwent two psychiatric hospitalizations, which were of short duration because insurance did not support an extended stay. On June 20, 2001, left alone with the five children (which was contrary to her doctor's orders), she systematically drowned them in the bathtub of her home. The baby was first and Noah, her oldest, was the last and the most difficult to subdue because he ran away and was strong enough to fight her. She repeatedly called the police, not explaining why, until they arrived to witness the catastrophic effects of her psychotic illness.

Yates was, in her mind, following Satan's directions. She believed her children had been tainted by the devil, and in her intense religious, delusional fervor, she was convinced that only death could guarantee them a place in heaven. She was also trying to provide them with a haven that they clearly did not have in her home. Those were the drivers, the purposes that filicide served for Andrea Yates.

A lack of awareness, absence of insight, which frequently accompanies delusional thinking, is typically seen as well in young people, girls and boys, with anorexia nervosa (see section "Anorexia Nervosa"). Their thinking is doggedly fixed. As bizarre as an idea may be,

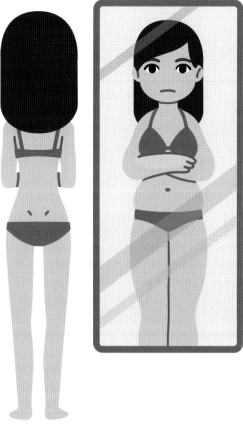

Anorexia nervosa.

like curing cancer, feeling fat weighing 81 pounds at 5 feet, 7 inches, or taking the life of a child to ensure its arrival in heaven, the person affected does not think it so at all. Their anger, avoidance, resistance, even assaultiveness directed toward others is the product of what they perceive is dismissal or interference by another person, family member, friend, caregiver, or stranger. Often, we hear from a person so affected, "I don't have a problem, except you!" Their behavior makes sense, but only from their perspective, not ours.

Oliver Sacks, the late neurologist and brilliant medical writer, commented in *The Man Who Mistook His Wife for a Hat and Other Clinical Tales*,

> It is not only difficult, it is impossible, for patients with certain right-hemisphere syndromes to know their own problems…And it is singularly difficult, for even the most sensitive observer, to picture the inner state, the 'situation', of such patients, for this is almost unimaginably remote from anything he himself has ever known. (Sacks 1985)

He was describing states of extreme denial as well as pinpointing its neurological locus in cases where the brain has been damaged. While there is significant evidence for changes in the brains of people with schizophrenia, the phenomena of delusions and denial have not been localized.

Anorexia Nervosa

Individuals with anorexia nervosa, which affects both girls and boys and women and men, have an intense fear of gaining weight. They are hungry just like the rest of us, think incessantly about food, but defy this basic demand of life. They selectively avoid certain foods, especially those high in fat. Their view of their bodies is blind to the emaciation that others see. Over time, if the disorder worsens, avoiding food and controlling weight becomes the centerpiece of their lives. The pleas of family are rejected; friends, school, and work are relegated to the margins of their lives.

Julia Kinney, a 17-year-old-high school junior, weighed in at 86 pounds, having lost another 6 pounds in the previous 2 weeks despite her outpatient treatment program, according to the pediatrician who had known her since she was a child. At 5 foot 6 inches (with a highest past weight of 120 pounds), she had entered a true danger zone, where disturbances in body potassium and other electrolytes can induce a potentially fatal cardiac arrhythmia. The pediatrician, in consultation with Julia's psychiatrist and family, arranged for emergency readmission to the psychiatric unit of a general hospital, where both her medical and mental health needs could be served.

As the nurses weighed Julia and took her vital signs (which were worrisome), she vigorously protested her hospitalization, despite looking like a starved victim of a prisoner of war camp. She wanted to go home and exercise and refused the juice and crackers offered to her saying, "I am fine." She had a severe case of anorexia nervosa, the restrictive (calorie limiting) type.

How can this type of behavior be purposeful? It is life-threatening, associated with a 20% lifetime rate of premature mortality from cardiac complications and suicide. It certainly is resolute, overriding hunger and self-preservation—but purposeful?

A number of illuminating studies on anorexia nervosa have been published in recent years by scientists at Columbia University and the New York State Psychiatric Institute. Their research has revealed that patients with this condition suffer severe anxiety, especially before a meal. This clinical research is not psychoanalytic work (which refers to understanding the underlying intrapsychic source of the anxiety), rather, it is phenomenological, that is, reporting on what exists, what can be observed and measured. And thus, it opens new avenues for therapeutics.

Patients with anorexia nervosa experience severe anxiety when they sit down to try to eat. This is not just feeling a little nervous; this is feeling an overwhelming state of fear, a panic, akin to your car suddenly skidding on ice and heading for a post on the side of the road. Such fear calls for, demands, getting away from the source of fear, getting away from (or not going to) the table, and, even more so, avoiding ingesting a morsel of food. Restrictive anorexia, the technical term for this type of not eating, is thus a way of managing severe anxiety—at a great price, of course.

The therapeutic implications of recent clinical research are, first, to appreciate the panic and dread patients with this condition experience and then to offer and provide treatment known to reduce this type of situation-bound anxiety. Researchers have shown that starvation worsens any existing anxiety (or other mood disturbance), so these patients experience more fear as they lose weight; conversely, as weight normalizes, their anxiety diminishes and their mood improves. One effective treatment technique is called exposure and response prevention: the person is exposed incrementally to the source of anxiety, and the response (running away, not eating) is gently blocked so that the anxiety is progressively overcome.

Of course, there are other necessary components in the treatment of anorexia nervosa, including life-saving electrolytes, programs for slow but progressive weight gain, and psychotherapy (especially cognitive-behavioral therapy) that focus on the disturbed body image and disturbed thinking that also occurs. Recent functional magnetic resonance imaging (fMRI) studies of the brain portray parts of the brain active in this disorder that are linked to habits, to the persistence of behaviors regardless of their consequences. But the essential element of therapeutic success, of saving lives, is reducing avoidance of food and encouraging restoration to a healthy weight.

———————————◆———————————

This first secret, that behavior serves a purpose, can sometimes only become visible when we suspend everyday logic. We have to look for more. We have to ask more, in a manner that allows a person to respond, over time, knowing that they will not be judged or harmed when allowing another person access to their private and sometimes previously inaccessible thinking.

I want to stress that understanding what drives behavior alone does not change it. The notion that "uncovering" an underlying feeling or motive, *abreacting* (releasing the underlying emotions), brings "cure" is very dated and deserves to remain so. But even if understanding does not by itself generate a cure, it does so much that is therapeutic: it replaces darkness with light, distortion with reason, blame with tolerance, dismissal with discussion, and powerlessness with problem solving.

References

Groves J: Taking care of the hateful patient. N Engl J Med 298(16):883–887, 1978 634331

Sacks O: The Man Who Mistook His Wife for a Hat and Other Clinical Tales. New York, Summit Books, 1985

Szasz T: The Myth of Mental Illness: Foundations of a Theory of Personal Conduct. New York, Hoeber-Harper, 1961

CHAPTER 2

THE POWER OF ATTACHMENT

Being deeply loved by someone
gives you strength,
while loving someone deeply
gives you courage.

Lao Tsu

The French film, *L'Enfant Sauvage* (*The Wild Child*, 1970), directed by François Truffaut, begins with a black and white screen that reads: "This story is authentic: it opens in 1798 in a French forest." We see a naked boy, prepubescent, in a forest in the Aveyron, a very rural Département in La France Profond (deepest France). A woman harvesting wild mushrooms spots him, runs away in fear, and finds some men to hunt him down. They use dogs to track his scent. They find his hiding hole, smoke him out, and capture him. He is feral and thrashes wildly against his captors. When alone, he rocks himself with the self-soothing behavior seen in children with autism.

The primitive child is without language. He is soon brought to Paris to a residential school for the "deaf and dumb," where he proves himself to be neither. But, he had lived a life without human attachment dating back to an uncertain time when he was very young. The consequences were painfully obvious. He was named Victor by the medical student who brought him into his home to raise and to attempt to civilize, with the help of a kindly housekeeper.

Three waves of psychological studies, from the 1920s to the 1960s, focused extensively on human attachments and the debilities that resulted from their absence. The first wave was led by Anna Freud (the youngest of Sigmund Freud's six children) and Melanie Klein, an Austrian-British analyst; the second by René Spitz; and the third by John Bowlby and Harry Harlow.

Anna Freud worked with children. She (like Melanie Klein, another psychoanalyst) helped lift psychoanalysis out of its preoccupation with

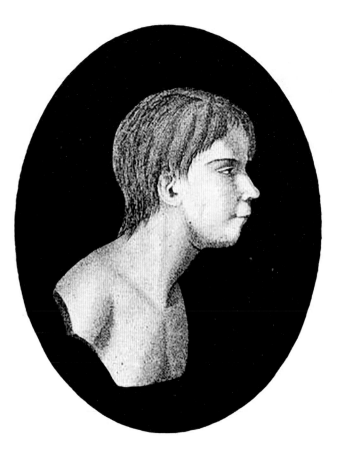

Der Wilde von Aveyron.

sex and aggression that her father, Sigmund, had promulgated. Anna emphasized the role of attachments to others (so-called objects, a term which worked then but is hardly an ideal term today to refer to human beings). World War II introduced Anna Freud to children deprived of their parents, and the need—when they were in foster care—to sustain close attachments to parental figures, even if they were not the biological parents. **Melanie Klein** is regarded as one of the founders of *object relations theory*, which holds that the early relationships in a child's environment are incorporated into the development of the psyche and fashion the future of his or her relationships and character.

René Spitz was an Austrian by birth, who moved to Paris, where he studied and practiced psychoanalysis, and then immigrated to the United States in 1939. He observed infants in foundling homes (orphanages) and discovered that when emotionally deprived because of the lack of maternal attention, these children developed what he called *anaclitic depression* (when the child becomes apathetic, listless, withdrawn, and disinterested in eating); anaclitic alludes to how an infant is emotionally propped up by the mother and figuratively falls over, actually becomes depressed, should she disappear. He also noted that if the "lost object" (namely, the mother or caretaker) was restored to the child within 5 months, there was still a chance of recovery. However, prolonging the deprivation beyond that time resulted in a state he termed "hospitalism," a deterioration in relationships and functioning that could be irrevocable.

The studies of **John Bowlby**, during World War II, of children who were thieves revealed that a good proportion had suffered early and prolonged separations from their mother or primary caregiver sometime during their first 5 years (Bowlby 1969). He too described the critical importance of a young child's caretaking environment and how lives can go awry if attachments are disrupted. Bowlby also emphasized the adverse, multigenerational impact on childhood development that resulted from the loss of attachment.

Harry Harlow, an American psychologist, is renowned for his rhesus macaque monkey studies. He subjected infant primates to maternal deprivation. Separated from their biological mothers, they were placed in a nursery with surrogates made from wire and wood, either bare or covered with cloth. He was able to show that the young macaques chose the cloth mother over the wire mother, even when the latter was a source of food. Contact—comfort—from a caregiver was, thus, a primary need that could override the need for food. Moreover, the cloth mothers became a basis for the capacity to explore, to seek change; they were also what the infants ran back to when subjected to fearful stimuli. Without the surrogate, the monkeys succumbed to fear, huddling and sucking their thumbs. It was the cloth surrogates, the soft blankies if you will, which provided security and were soothing for the stressed macaques. In later experiments, Harlow demonstrated the consequences for monkeys isolated from caregivers for 6 months, namely, they became debilitated, and 12 months of isolation destroyed their social capacities. Notably, by demonstrating that there is a critical time for forming attachments, he showed that monkeys isolated for a comparable period of time in later life did not experience the same adverse effects. In other words, attachment and normal social development are achieved early and provide a foundation for life, when a child's environment includes that opportunity (Suomi and Leroy 1982).

These brief sketches of these great investigators into human development cannot do justice to the breadth and value of their work or to their influence on many other gifted psychologically oriented practitioners and researchers. But even such a limited glance gives us a basis for appreciating the power of attachment, of human (object) relationships and how they serve as the soil in which the members of the human community are rooted. It is the power of attachment that fashions our personalities, underlies many of our motivations, and explains a host of our behaviors.

When my son was about 1 year old, he selected from among a heap of stuffed animals, blankets, and other cuddly items a rabbit hand puppet, gray with white markings and about a foot long, to be his constant companion. We called him rabbit-rabbit. He (the rabbit) was dragged about everywhere and of course slept bunched up against my son's cheek.

While not every child has a cuddly companion (and some suck their thumbs instead or as well), it is more common than not. Child psychologists call these transitional objects, a term conceived by **D.W. Winnicott**, a British pediatrician and analyst whose work gained prominence and influence in the 1930s. Winnicott believed that the transitional object served a critical role for children up to 3 years of age when they begin to separate from their primary caregiver, their mother. Early attachment is so powerful he concluded that the child needs a way of tolerating separation from mother, a necessary developmental step in all our lives. The transitional object, the rabbit in my son's case, enables a young child to be without his or her mother yet not panic at being alone. You can see how blankies (as well as stuffed animals and the like) came to be called security blankets and how some adults even adopt a similar such item (like a scarf or T-shirt) that continues to serve the same comforting function.

When my son was about 4, and still carrying the now very ragged rabbit, we accidentally left it in a taxi. Upon discovering its loss later that day (it was I who did—not my son), I was in a state. I called every taxi company and labored to find it. I was more upset than my son! We did not find it. I finally quieted down, and my son seemed to never look back.

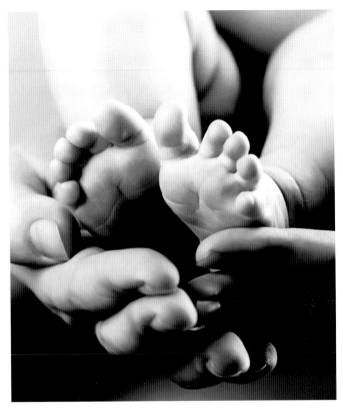

Infancy.

Attachment Theories and Styles

Theories about attachment posit that as individuals we vary in our early predispositions to the caretakers in our lives (like mothers or other primary parental figures). The child encounters his or her world of primary caregivers, some of whom can help to foster a sense of safety and security and some do the contrary because of emotional unpredictability, indifference, or actual physical harm or cruelty. Temperament and exposure, nature and nurture, shape the child's inner emotional states and capacity to regulate them.

Children thus develop varied styles of attachment, which reflect what inner emotional security or lack of it they have established. The two principal styles of attachment are called secure and insecure, and they can be recognized as early as 1 year of age. The child's attachment style will determine how he or she responds to the challenges of development, including the ability to be alone, the facility to act with some confidence in relationships and self-expression, and the capacity for intimacy with others. Early insecurity becomes ingrained and persists into adulthood if there are no experiences to alter it.

Secure attachments in adults are marked by a person's capacity to put into perspective disappointments, frustrations, separations, and minor traumas. People with secure attachments are resilient to life's slings and arrows. They have the ability to be emotionally close to others, to be intimate with others, and to permit themselves both to depend upon others and be responsibly dependable themselves.

Insecure attachments manifest in three principal forms, although more than one form can exist in any individual.

Individuals with *dismissive/avoidant* behavioral styles tend to distance themselves from others. They do not seem to place significant value on relationships, and they have a type of faux independence that can make them appear strong—at least on the surface. When reliable information about their early lives can be obtained, there is often evidence of parental neglect or rejection.

Individuals who are *preoccupied* and/or *anxious* are highly focused on their relationships and whether they can depend on them, as well as how others may see them (and thus treat them). They are unable to reflect on and learn from their past experiences with others; they tend to remain connected to and reliant on parents and others who served in caregiving roles in their lives. They can seem emotionally starved, desperate for connection, and given to acting in dependent, child-like ways.

Individuals who are *disorganized* have the greatest problems with adult relationships. Like Karen Anderson (described below), they can be dramatic and unstable in their relationships. Many with this form of insecure attachment suffered early trauma (abuse or neglect) or loss of parents, home, or safety (e.g., forced refugees). The insecurity leads to intense, abortive relationships, as illustrated in Karen's story, and at times desperate, self-destructive efforts to maintain contact. Their problems often echo through generations, with the insecure child becoming a troubled mother to her child.

Karen Anderson was 20 when I was asked to consult with her. She was a patient on a psychiatric ward of a general hospital. She had cut her wrists after her boyfriend left her. Intellectually gifted and creative, she had a stormy adolescence with early alcohol and drug use, impulsive and risky behaviors (including going to sketchy clubs late at night, picking up strangers, and having unprotected sex), and angry outbursts when she felt she was not "getting enough" from her parents, friends, or in the transient relationships she had with young and older men.

Her moods were as varied as what has been said about Chicago: If you don't like the weather, wait 5 minutes. Minor frustrations produced dramatic tears and tantrums when the need for immediate and continuous contact was not met by whomever she was attached to, often in a clingy way. When she met someone she was drawn to, Karen leapt into an emotional relationship, which was usually of quite brief duration because of her unbearable neediness (and because she could not tolerate actual intimacy or a mutually rewarding relationship; in fact, what she needed was to be cared for). This pattern of neediness and an inability to be satisfied traced back to when she was a little girl, her foster parents reported.

Drives and Higher Needs

In psychology, drive theory holds that humans, and other living creatures, are born with certain inherent needs. These include satisfying hunger, self-preservation, sex (procreation), attachment, exploration, and some say aggression. When a drive (sometimes synonymous with an instinct) is not satisfied, a person, or animal, enters a state of physical and psychological disequilibrium, which can be felt as distress and which presses for whatever action is needed to reduce the distress and return to a state of equilibrium (or put more positively, to a state of relief or even satisfaction).

Drives operate automatically and are more or less universal within a species (although there can be individual exceptions in a diverse world). There is no training needed to learn to express these drives, but significantly, any number of learning theorists and social psychologists assert that as we progress through the mammalian chain to primates, instincts can be modified by experience and training.

Abraham Maslow's hierarchy of human needs exemplifies the developmental progression from foundational basic instincts or drives to higher-order human needs. When our most fundamental needs for

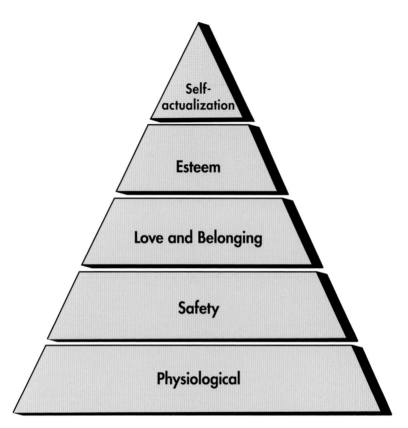

Maslow's hierarchy of needs.

food, shelter, and safety are realized, Maslow believed that humans can mature and fulfill higher-order needs such as love and belonging (attachment), self-esteem, and the capacity for self-actualization (to experience competence and worthiness). Whereas behaviorists, dating back to the early work of B.F. Skinner, may explain these higher-order needs in other ways, what matters is that as the primate and then human cerebral cortex evolved, our basic drives came under (to greater or lesser degrees) its control. Neurological case studies in which there is damage to the cortex, especially the frontal lobes, reveal how more basic, primitive drives without cortical control become unfettered and can render a person impulsive, aggressive, voracious, and sexually unconstrained.

The matrix for human development, even for learned behavior, is an interpersonal relationship. We learn, we grow, and we surpass our basic drives and self-absorbed behaviors in the milieu of and through human relations. Here is where attachment comes in and demonstrates its power.

Primacy of Attachment Over Drives

The instinct or drive for self-preservation is perhaps as early and fundamental a force as exists in human nature. Yet it is hardly absolute. Self-preservation can be subordinated to other needs, especially the need for attachment—attachments that can be seen in examples as varied as the mother-child bond, destructive relationships, and heroic acts.

All of us who have been witnesses to a birth and to the moments that ensue appreciate how that infant now has a protector who will sacrifice her life for the safety of her child. Of course, there are instances where this is not the case, where that bond does not form because of the limitations or psychopathology of the mother, but few rules don't have some rare exception (or include deviance). Typically, however, a physiological and psychological event occurs whereby the mother's attachment to her child supersedes her own self-interests, including her self-preservation. The rupture through death or unwanted separation of a mother's attachment to a child thus evokes an almost inconsolable grief and heartbreaking agony.

Luisa Caper appeared for her third visit that year to an urban emergency department bleeding from facial wounds and a likely broken arm. She was 29 years old, the mother of a 1-year-old daughter (who was being cared for by her grandmother), and a waitress in a chain restaurant. For the past several years, on and off, she lived with Frank, the father of her child and an unemployed man in his late 30s who was a binge drinker. His drinking, however, had become more frequent, and when under the influence, he was an angry, aggressive drunk, especially to Ms. Caper. She never pressed charges against him and more so never insisted he get out of her home. At each emergency department visit, the nursing and medical staff always introduced her to social workers, who tried to help her protect herself through an order of protection or through temporary and safe housing designed particularly for battered women. But she repeatedly, if ashamedly, did not take them up on their offers.

In my work, I have met battered women, victims of domestic violence (beaten and traumatized children too, but that is another matter that will be touched on in Chapter 4, "Chronic Stress Is the Enemy"). Many cities and counties have developed special programs and services to assist these women in exiting the grip of perilous attachment to abusive men. At times, victims of violence (and they can be men and youth as well) respond with violence, and they become involved with the correctional system, which is of course no solution. The attachment of abused women to their abuser, however, many times overrides their safety and sometimes puts them at mortal risk. They can succeed in breaking free from the abusive relationship, but it usually takes time and developing the capacity to seek a different way of meeting their emotional needs.

Linda Mills' remarkable work, including her book *Violent Partners*, offers many insights into who enters and cannot leave violent relationships (Mills 2008). She points to early lives with unstable caregivers and attachments, which also may account for the multigenerational nature of this problem. Additional problems in relationships, especially with other family and friends, leave these troubled people with no sense of group or community, which is essential to believing that there are other ways to live and people to turn to. She writes about shame in those who expose themselves to violence, which can leave a person with the feeling "I don't deserve any better." She refers to this phenomenon as "damage seeking damage." There is even the paradoxical experience of enduring abuse as a means of demonstrating a form of connection and loyalty that serves the victim's needs for pride and self-respect, not just attachment. Finally, certain cultures either explicitly or implicitly support subordination and abuse especially of women as socially acceptable; these cultures can create pariahs of those who try to escape the cycle of subjugation and violence.

An appreciation of each and all of the forces at work in violent attachments, ones that subordinate safety to maintain an attachment, leads to an awareness of the complexity of this problem and emphasizes how solutions must respond to the multiple forces at work to break such "fierce attachments." At the very least, new and safe relationships and community are needed for a person to realize that respect and mutual gratification can be achieved by pursuing a path away from violence.

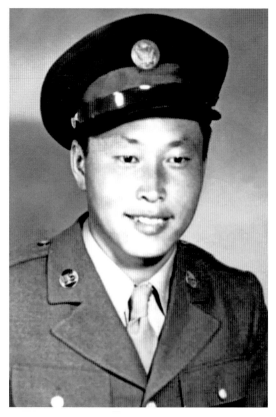

Private Sakato.

On June 21, 2000, President Bill Clinton awarded George Sakato the Medal of Honor, our nation's highest award for valor.[1] Private Sakato served in World War II as an infantryman. In combat in the fall of 1944, his squad was besieged by German gunfire. Under heavy attack, Sakato killed five enemy combatants and captured four others. Despite his diminutive stature (he was 5 feet 4 inches tall), on his own he rushed a hilltop stronghold enabling his fellow soldiers to destroy the site. When his squad leader was killed in the ongoing battle, Sakato continued to place himself in mortal danger, killing another seven enemy soldiers and assisting in the capture of many others.

Heroes may not be common, yet they regularly appear, especially in war. They also valiantly appear in disasters and other emergencies. What characterizes them is their capacity to place the lives and the interests of others before their own need for preservation and safety. It is not glory that drives this type of heroism, though glory may be one of its rewards (although we often hear an authentic hero say he or she was "just doing my job"). The drive that explains the capacity to overcome mortal danger is the bond to others, an attachment to a "brother," a fellow soldier, a team, a family, a community, and even a nation. While not everyone can overcome the instinctive need to flee, to survive, the examples we witness and read about and admire are testaments to the power of attachment.

---

[1]By the way, Private Sakato did receive a Distinguished Service Cross after his heroic actions. He was recommended for the Medal of Honor also, but he did not receive it because of his Japanese ancestry and the fact that we were at war with Japan. President Clinton made that right—awarding him his due honor at the White House, along with 21 other Asian Americans, 15 posthumously.

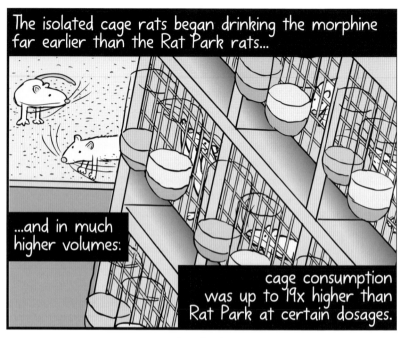

Rat Park

Addictions and the Power of Attachment

Psychologist Bruce Alexander developed in the 1970s what came to be called the Rat Park experiment (Alexander et al. 1981). Previous studies of rats had demonstrated that when a rat was put in a cage alone with two water bottles—one filled with water and the other with heroin or cocaine—the rat would repetitively drink from the drug-laced bottle until it overdosed and died. Alexander wondered: Is this the result of the drug or the setting? He put rats in "rat parks," where they were among others and free to roam and play, with access to the same two types of bottles. Remarkably, the rat park rodents preferred the plain water, and when they did imbibe from the drug-filled bottle they did so intermittently, not obsessively, and never overdosed. Attachment and social community beat the power of drugs.

Norman Zinberg, M.D., a former colleague at Cambridge Hospital in Massachusetts, was tasked during the Vietnam War with investigating the high rates of heroin (and other drug) use among soldiers deployed to the war. One in five soldiers on duty in Vietnam was regularly using heroin (Zinberg 1984). There was great concern within the U.S. Army not just about this drug use but also about what would happen when these soldiers returned home. Would they go into withdrawal? Would they continue to use and destroy their family relationships and their prospects for a future? Would they resort to criminal activities to fund a drug habit? Dr. Zinberg said no. Upon return, he predicted that this group of men would have no greater rates of drug addiction than the general (nonmilitary) population. He was right. Their families, communities, and other attachments prevailed, and they left their drug use in the jungle where the horrific circumstances of terror and deadly combat were the "cage" that fostered their use of drugs. They no longer needed to rely on drugs to tolerate the setting they were in, and they built a life free of drug abuse once again (Zinberg 1984).

Therapeutic Alliance

The therapeutic alliance is one of the most important, yet often overlooked, aspects of psychotherapy, counseling, and even general medical care. At the heart of the therapeutic alliance is the patient's trust that the doctor or counselor has the patient's interests in mind: that the patient's needs truly come first, not those of the professional or institution providing care.

A clinician, physician, or other professional must earn the trust of a patient. For some patients, that trust can come early; it is based on their past experience of people who cared for them without exploiting them. Other patients have lived a life in which early and important caregivers were unstable or narcissistically self-absorbed, making development of trusting relationships either largely impossible or fraught with doubt. Still other patients have serious mental disorders in which paranoia colors their perceptions and makes trust highly elusive.

Some mental health professionals and doctors have what can seem like an innate capacity to foster trust in their patients. I am not talking about psychopaths who engender trust but do so falsely and manipulatively. I mean the kind of caregiver we all want—someone whom we experience as trustworthy, putting our interests above his or her own, above his or her convenience or profit or the rigid demands of the bureaucracy in which they work. A hallmark of these professionals is that their patients return for appointments. Moreover, the mental health clinicians and physicians (in all branches of medicine) who are experienced as trustworthy, as likeable, by their patients are far less likely to be sued, even if they were negligent in their provision of care.

Medical liability cases are usually a blend of bad outcomes and the bad feelings generated when a doctor does not seem to care about the patient or behaves in cold and evasive ways.

When I was in psychiatric training, I learned that one of the best predictors of outcome in the psychotherapy that I would provide was whether a therapeutic alliance had been developed and maintained. Those patients who experienced a strong therapeutic relationship would tend to do better in "love and work" (the principal aims of therapy, a reference often attributed to Freud). I would need to be alert to those moments in my work with patients when the alliance was at risk, from events in the patient's life or times when therapy was not helping. The work of understanding and repairing a rupture in the alliance could not only restore the emotional safety necessary for psychotherapy, but it could create moments of what has been called a corrective emotional experience. That's when, in many a relationship, the challenges to trust are stirred up and an honest inquiry into what happened enables its restoration.

What is the source of the therapeutic alliance? At the risk of over-simplifying, it is the capacity for attachment, for developing a healthy bond with another person that is the foundation, the soil, for the trust needed for an alliance. From that soil can grow the ability of a person to put himself or herself in the hands of another person, to take the risks and to sustain the work needed for productive psychotherapy. I imagine it is not unlike when a child is ready for his or her parent to let go of the bicycle for the first time; the child trusts and dares to go free and be autonomous. Achieving a healthy, trusting attachment in mental health treatment, as well as in medical care, thus needs to be a goal in itself for the clinician/doctor–patient relationship. Part of the cure lies in and derives from the sustained capacity to trust the caregiver, when it is genuinely earned. That's the power of the attachment, and that's why the therapeutic alliance is a good predictor of clinical outcome.

Managing Our Emotions

My friend and colleague at Columbia, Dr. Deborah Cabaniss, a professor and author, writes about attachment in her book about psychotherapy (Cabaniss et al. 2013). She points out that the attachment styles mentioned earlier in this chapter are often passed on from parent to child. Our capacity for secure attachment may offer us resilience in the face of everyday slings and arrows as well as when we face even more disruptive traumas and losses.

All children and adults must develop the capacity to manage their emotions, including fear, insecurity, doubt, anxiety, excitement, and frustration. This capacity, often called *affect regulation*, is instrumental to functioning in relationships, in school, in work, and even in play. Those youths who begin with insecure attachments are often limited in their ability to regulate these feelings and thus to proceed with healthy emotional and interpersonal development. A faulty foundation may breed problems in living, which, in turn, reinforce insecurity and compound the frailties a person may have.

Signs of poor affect regulation, one of the potential consequences of insecure attachment, include labile moods, impulsivity, poor self-esteem, and identity problems. *Empathy*, the capacity to appreciate how others see themselves and the world, is also compromised and undermines the achievement of mutual, caring relationships.

The insecure attachment of the child can be seen and felt years later in the actions of the adult. For example, a parent whose early life was beset with inconsistency or abuse, who did not form critical strong bonds with caregivers may fear change and loss and be too restrictive with his or her children, stifling their quest for independence and autonomy and impairing his or her own family relationships.

   We can expect that this patient will also live out his insecure attachment in psychotherapy, which will permit an opportunity for him to understand his reactions, create new narratives (about himself), and work to achieve more secure attachments with his family and others in his life. The therapeutic experience is in itself a microcosm, an interpersonal opportunity for insight and the creation of new, more secure attachments to the therapist and then to the important people who populate a person's life. Those changes in attachment, step by step, enable more effective regulation of feelings, which, in turn, build an even stronger and more secure attachment style. A similar process, though one that will likely be more tumultuous and protracted, could occur in a successful treatment for Karen, the young woman described earlier in this chapter.

What Makes for a Good Life

In 1938, a research study began at Harvard College, enrolling 268 college sophomores and then a few years later 456 young men from Boston's inner city living in underprivileged neighborhoods and circumstances. The Harvard Study of Adult Development continues today.

   Some of the original research subjects, privileged Harvard undergraduate men, many of whom went on to become professionals and successful businessmen and one who became a president of the United States, were entered into an ongoing study of their lives. The young men from the inner city were added to create a comparison group. The aim of the study was to answer this question: How can we live a long and happy life?

   Robert Waldinger, M.D., the study's current director and a professor at Harvard Medical School (who succeeded George Vaillant, M.D.), continues to ask the study participants what makes them happier and healthier (Waldinger 2015). The answers are not money and fame. They are the ongoing presence of good relationships with spouses, family, and friends. It turns out that quality relationships, even those that have their conflicts but are characterized by a deep sense that the other person is there for them—that they can truly depend on the other person if and when needed—are protective. Those with quality relationships lived longer and even had better cognitive functioning (as measured by memory tests). Unwelcome isolation and loneliness as well as high-conflict relationships were toxic, at least to the men in this study. Loneliness kills, a finding replicated in a multitude of sociological studies. Loneliness, by the way is different from *solitude*, a chosen state of being alone, which can be for some a very rewarding lifestyle.

Women were also studied in the Harvard longitudinal study, which included them later. For women, it was learned that greater security in relationships predicted better memory and well-being (Waldinger et al. 2015).

The power of attachment keeps making its case. If we want to add life to our years rather than simply more years to our lives, we can succeed by attending to what makes us human, namely, our healthy connections with those we love and honor. The implication for our professional efforts, as well, for mental health and medical care is clear: to enable those who seek help (and sometimes those who do not) to live happier and healthier lives (see Fries 1980).

References

Alexander BK, Beyerstein BL, Hadaway PF, Coambs RB: Effect of early and later colony housing on oral ingestion of morphine in rats. Pharmacol Biochem Behav 58(4):571–576, 1981 7291261

Bowlby J: Attachment and Loss, 2nd Edition, Vol 1: Attachment. New York, Basic Books, 1969

Cabaniss DL, Cherry S, Douglas CJ, et al: Psychodynamic Formulation. Hoboken, NJ, Wiley-Blackwell, 2013

Fries JF: Aging, natural death, and the compression of morbidity. N Engl J Med 303(3):130–135, 1980 7383070

Mills LG: Violent Partners: A Breakthrough Plan for Ending the Cycle of Abuse. New York, Basic Books, 2008

Suomi JS, Leroy HA: In memoriam: Harry F. Harlow (1905–1981). Am J Primatol 2:319–342, 1982

Waldinger RJ: "The Good Life," TEDx video, 15:03. Posted November 30, 2015. Available at: https://www.youtube.com/watch?v=q-7zAkwAOYg&feature=youtu.be

Waldinger RJ, Cohen S, Schulz MS, Crowell JA: Security of attachment to spouses in late life: concurrent and prospective links with cognitive and emotional wellbeing. Clin Psychol Sci 3(4):516–529 2015 26413428

Zinberg NE: Drug, Set, and Setting: The Basis for Controlled Intoxicant Use. New Haven, CT, Yale University Press, 1984

CHAPTER 3

AS A RULE, LESS IS MORE

There is nothing men will not do,
there is nothing they have not done,
to recover their health…They have
submitted to be half-drowned in water,
and half-choked with gases, to be buried
up to their chins in earth, to be seared
with hot irons like galley-slaves,
to be crimped with knives, like cod-fish,
to have needles thrust into their flesh,
and bonfires kindled on their skin,
to swallow all sorts of abominations,
and to pay for all this, as if to be singed
and scalded were costly privilege,
as if blisters were a blessing,
and leeches were a luxury.

Oliver Wendell Holmes

In sections of southern France, many a church displays a statue of a saint pulling up his robe to reveal a skin lesion (a bubo) on his thigh. A dog stands by his side, typically offering a piece of bread held in its mouth. This Catholic figure, Saint Roch, is generally not well known elsewhere, unless you watched the film *The Godfather Part II*, in which he is displayed in a procession through New York City's Little Italy.

Saint Roch, known as a protector against contagious diseases, was born at the end of the thirteenth century in Montpellier to the wife of the governor of that city. On the death of his parents, when he was 20, he gave away all his worldly goods to the poor and began life as an itinerant pilgrim. But it was during the epidemic of the bubonic plague that St. Roch found his calling. He moved about among public hospitals in plague-ridden cities in Italy, reportedly effecting cures by his touch.

Soon, however, he fell ill with the plague. Upon being expelled because he was ill from the town in Italy where he had wandered, he isolated himself in a nearby forest, where he reportedly cured himself by simple living and the help of prayer. A dog belonging to a local huntsman came upon St. Roch and is said to have brought him bread each day so he would not starve.

St. Roch's career as a healer was cut short when he returned to Montpellier. He was arrested and jailed as a spy, and unable to cure unjust incarceration, he languished in prison until his death 5 years later. It was his healing work, which did not call for excesses of intervention but rather simple care and belief, which earned him a place in the pantheon of saints.

First, Do No Harm

When a disease defies efforts at cure, because it is not well understood or its therapeutics remains limited or rudimentary, there is a powerful human tendency to up the ante. Do more, do something radical, take unusual measures to effect improvement are among the human drives to be reckoned with because they provide help infrequently and often have unwanted and problematic effects. *Primum non nocere*, first, do no harm, is the first law of medicine. It is unfortunately a law that is violated more than the speed limit in most states. For psychiatry and mental health, general medical care as well, being able to do less is a secret that has been eclipsed by too many heroic efforts to do more. **As a rule, less is more.**

Medications

Susan Long was a rising star in her profession in her late 20s when she came to see me in my office at the Massachusetts General Hospital in the late 1970s. As she earned greater advancement and success, she grew more anxious and afraid to leave her home. Her anxiety became so severe that it threatened her job and totally shut down time with friends and dating. I recommended a course of psychotherapy to work on what might be underlying problems stirred up by her achievements and medication treatment in light of the severity of her symptoms and the risk they posed for her livelihood.

This was a decade before Prozac and the other serotonin-enhancing drugs that I would be able to prescribe. Tranquilizers like Librium and Valium were around, but neither Ms. Long nor I was keen on employing them because of their often troublesome effects on mental clarity and wakefulness, as well as the susceptibility of our bodies to become dependent on benzodiazepines. Tricyclic antidepressants were available (like imipramine), but they had a host of lousy side effects (like blurred vision, dry mouth, and constipation) and were not all that effective for the symptoms she had. However, there was a class of drugs, monoamine oxidase inhibitors (MAOIs), then far more popular than today, which I was familiar with and suggested she try. I explained these types of medications and their potential risks and benefits to her. I said that perhaps over time therapy would help, but her concerns about imminent job loss because of her dysfunction made Ms. Long want to start on a medication, at least for now.

I wrote a prescription for Nardil, one 15-mg pill twice a day, increasing to three times a day on day four after she started this medication. We scheduled a meeting for the following week to begin therapy and review how she was doing with the medication. Late on the fifth day after she began taking the drug, she left me a phone message asking to speak with me as soon as possible. I promptly called and found her at home. "Doctor," she said, "I had to crawl to the phone because if I stand up, I'll surely pass out!" She was experiencing *postural hypotension*, a big drop in her blood pressure when she stood up and a side effect of Nardil. I had made her worse before she stood a chance of feeling better.

I explained what was happening and how to manage the symptoms (a lot of fluids, a little salt, and rising to a standing position very slowly) until her blood level of the drug naturally diminished by simply not taking any more. That worked. But Ms. Long was very reluctant to resume the Nardil and stay on it for the weeks needed to see its potential beneficial effects. I was concerned that I had caused problems that would interfere with recovering from debilitating anxiety and keeping her job!

But she was a trooper, and I had gained some of her trust. A week later, she resumed taking Nardil but only one 15-mg pill/day; we monitored her response very carefully and increased the dose when she felt comfortable doing so. It took a bit longer, but she got to 45 mg/day and began to notice reductions in her anxiety and improvements in her ability to leave home, to be at work and among her colleagues, and to socialize.

That was an important lesson for me, and one that physicians (and now prescribing nurses) have to learn: *start low, go slow* when it comes to many a medication. Less was more for Ms. Long until she could tol-

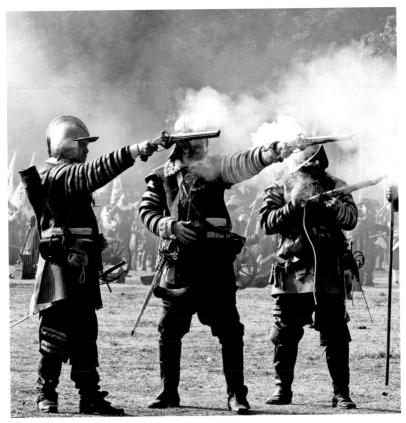

Sixteenth-century battlefield.

erate more and derive a therapeutic effect and thus not abandon a treatment that would work for her.

Psychotherapy

This same principle of less is more can apply to psychotherapy as well.

In 1986, my good friend and colleague Dr. Bob Drake and I published a pair of articles on the "negative" effects of intensive psychological treatments of schizophrenia (Drake and Sederer 1986a, 1986b). We used as a metaphor surgical wound healing.

Ancient Egyptian doctors understood, and inscribed on papyrus dating back to 1700 B.C., that wounds did best when debris was removed, when they were gently washed with water, and when they were covered to allow natural healing. Less was more. But in the fourteenth century, the ancient ninth-century Chinese invention, which would cause more damage than about anything else man-made up until that time, became more widely implemented in Western warfare: gunpowder. Men were shooting one another at a brisk rate. To treat gunshot wounds, which frequently become infected, surgeons employed far more aggressive means of treating wounded soldiers: they poured boiling oil into their wounds. The results were, as you can imagine, disastrous. However, this barbaric practice did not end until 200 years later when a French army surgeon rediscovered the gentle and simple care of wounds—but only after he ran out of oil. A destructive tide had been turned back, fortunately, and the idea that less is more again prevailed. Gentle cleaning and protection resumed being, after two centuries of horrific treatment, the standard of wound care and has remained so today.

Schizophrenia affects about 1% of the world's population. It usually has an onset in adolescence or early adulthood, with psychotic symptoms of hallucinations and delusions appearing at the outset, accompanied by social withdrawal, severe anxiety, and loss of everyday functioning at school, home, and work. In recent years, psychiatry has rediscovered that people with this serious mental illness can improve over time, even if they still have residual symptoms of the condition. Recovery, healing, is possible but requires that treatments not aggravate a person's mental state or drive them away from the prudent, gentle care that can make a valuable difference in their lives.

In our articles (Drake and Sederer 1986a, 1986b), we reported on how intensive psychotherapy (delivered either too frequently or in an emotionally confrontational, unstructured, or deeply explorative fashion) can produce unnecessary and overwhelming psychic stimulation in vulnerable patients and induce regression, including further loss of reality testing and functional capability. Group therapies that are provocative—that urge the expression of anger and other intense feelings or evoke excessive self-disclosure—can also be toxic to people with impaired cognitive functioning and confusion about boundaries relating to themselves and others. Family therapy, too, that invites expression of conflict and feelings or is blaming or judgmental (of patient or family) has negative effects on the mental state and the course of illness of people with schizophrenia.

Instead, practical, problem-solving therapies are helpful, as are psychoeducation and providing self-management and social skills training. These are the gentle, less is more approaches that allow for improved functioning and a path to recovery in people with this serious mental disorder.

Early-Onset Psychosis

One hundred thousand, approximately, teenagers and young adults, male and female, of every class, ethnicity, and race in the United States annually experience the first onset of a non-drug-induced psychotic illness, like schizophrenia and schizoaffective disorder (the latter being a disorder in which psychotic symptoms are present in addition to serious mood problems).

Until recently, if a young person became psychotic, it was commonplace that years went by before their condition, even if it was obvious to those around them, was recognized and properly diagnosed and the individual received some form of psychiatric treatment. Delays such as this (referred to as duration of untreated psychosis) have been shown to be highly associated with a more severe course of illness and greater disability over a lifetime.

For those who found treatment (or, more likely, their families found it for them), the convention has been the prescription of high doses of antipsychotic medications and a long wait for a case manager at a mental health clinic where others with more advanced stages of psychotic illness would come for their medication or monitoring. Few youths could tolerate the sedation, muscle tightness, and restlessness that high doses of antipsychotic medications produced, especially in young men. Witnessing the chronicity in patients who were decades older was alarming and repellent to their self-image and hopes. The absence of a program aimed at recovery was anathema. It was no wonder few returned for services, ironically fating them to exactly what they and their families feared the most: a life lost to illness.

However, preceding the introduction of early psychosis treatment programs in the United States, countries such as Australia (led by the Australian of the year in 2010, Dr. Patrick McGorry), the United Kingdom, and Denmark had already been at work providing a dramatically different approach to early-onset psychotic illnesses. And now, in the United States, new programs such as NAVIGATE and OnTrackNY, led by Dr. John Kane (at Northwell Health) and my gifted

Natural History of Schizophrenia
Rationale for Early Detection and Intervention

Stages of Illness

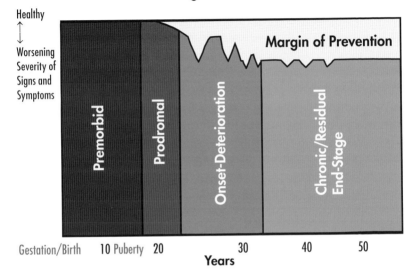

Duration of untreated psychosis and later disability.

Adapted from Lewis and Lieberman 2000.

colleague Dr. Lisa Dixon (at the New York State Psychiatric Institute and Columbia University), respectively, are changing the trajectory and preventing disability in those youths who become ill with psychosis. These are programs trying to help young people recover and have lives they might otherwise have been denied.

Under the rubric of Recovery After an Initial Schizophrenia Episode (RAISE), a research initiative of the National Institute of Mental Health, or the coordinated specialty care program (CSC), a recovery-oriented treatment program specifically addressing first-episode psychosis, both NAVIGATE and OnTrackNY were introduced to eschew the conventional care of psychosis, namely, too much medication and too little else. Less medication can be more when it is provided in natural settings, with the support of families, and with special attention from educational and vocational specialists to keep youths in school or work and put them on a path to the normative goals of young adulthood. It is not that RAISE and CSC are antimedication; we know that relapse is highly likely unless people take antipsychotic medications early in the illness of schizophrenia. However, modest doses and careful attention to minimizing any uncomfortable side effects informs prescribing practices. In addition, stress-reducing and health-promoting practices like meditation, yoga, exercise, healthful diet, and nutraceuticals are recognized as welcome allies, not odd practices to be scoffed at.

In his blog, the Director of the National Institutes of Health Dr. Francis Collins wrote the following:

> A great example is the Simpson family, which lives just outside of Lansing, MI. At age 17, son Collin was hospitalized to work through his first psychosis, receiving what his father Tom describes as "generic care." When Collin was released from the hospital, Tom says he felt utterly unprepared to arrange the aftercare and take steps to reduce risk

As a Rule, Less Is More

of a relapse. He tried to find a psychiatrist in Lansing for his son, but he couldn't locate one who was available to see new patients. That's when Tom's sister, who worked in community mental health, suggested that Collin enroll in NAVIGATE.

Tom calls NAVIGATE's individualized, team-based approach "a godsend." Collin not only received timely psychiatric care and careful monitoring of his medications, he also got help to prepare and pass his General Educational Development (GED) test, guidance in drafting his resume, and assistance in finding a job. Meanwhile, Tom and other members of the family participated in the NAVIGATE educational program and got their questions answered about psychosis, schizophrenia, and what they should and shouldn't expect from Collin. "We would have been clueless if they hadn't brought us all in as a group," Tom says. "It was a critical part." (Collins 2015)

I like to think of early psychosis treatment programs as characterized by less reliance on medication, less neglect, less distancing from family, and less clinic- and hospital-based care. Less is replaced by a more comprehensive set of services delivered at homes, community centers, playgrounds, and even McDonald's and a resilient, recovery-oriented view of the future. Less medication and monitoring is more when *comprehensive treatment* aligns with what the person under care is age appropriately seeking. In these ways, less becomes a lot more. What's more, so to speak, over time, RAISE and CSC programs may not even require more money if costly hospital and emergency services are reduced, as we are already seeing in the programs underway in New York State. In time, we may also see reductions in criminal justice, shelter, and welfare costs as well. Less money spent unnecessarily for crisis services leaves more for school, rehabilitation, and recovery.

Less can be more when the treatment that is delivered discards practices of limited effectiveness and with too many adverse consequences but only when complemented by comprehensive services—

where *necessary services are coupled with sufficient services*—including those based on the goals of recovery and provided in ways and in settings where those served are comfortable and are willing to engage. That's a secret worth spreading.

Clinical Antipsychotic Trials of Intervention Effectiveness (CATIE)

In 2001, the National Institute of Mental Health launched the largest federally funded study ever of psychiatric medications, the Clinical Antipsychotic Trials of Intervention Effectiveness (CATIE). Its purpose was to compare the older, so-called first-generation antipsychotic medications, with the newer second-generation drugs.

Nearly 1,500 patients, ages 18–65 years, with schizophrenia were enrolled in this study at 57 clinical sites in the United States. Perphenazine (Trilafon) was used as the first-generation agent (to represent others of its vintage like haloperidol, chlorpromazine, and fluphenazine). Olanzapine (Zyprexa), risperidone (Risperdal), quetiapine (Seroquel), and ziprasidone (Geodon) were the second-generation agents used; they were assigned randomly, and appeared as identical-looking capsules, to study participants. At the time, all of these second-generation antipsychotics were drugs under patent protection and were vastly more expensive than the generic perphenazine. A second phase of the study sought to examine those patients who discontinued medication because it did not work or because the side effects were intolerable; in this circumstance, another medication, clozapine (Clozaril), was added to the roster of agents prescribed (Lieberman and Stroup 2011; Swarz et al. 2008).

The results of the CATIE studies, published in more than 80 scientific articles, a book, and many commentaries, were, first, astounding in what they revealed and, second, had dreadfully little impact on practice.

The most disturbing finding, which actually did not surprise most clinicians who treat people with schizophrenia, was the incredibly high rate—74% of patients (ranging from 64% to 82% depending on the drug)—at which the study participants stopped taking the medication prescribed. Many patients continued in the study taking a different medication, suggesting that the problem was not noncompliance. While opinions vary, there is a general view that stopping medication was the result of the limited effectiveness of a given drug as well as its troubling side effects.

Medication nonadherence, patients not continuing to take what is prescribed, is a very familiar problem to practicing mental health clinicians and to the loved ones of people with schizophrenia and other serious mental disorders. First, as mentioned, patients tend not to like the side effects of the medications, which can be very different from first- to second-generation antipsychotics. The former are notorious for producing *akathisia*, a feeling of awful restlessness that can get so bad that there are reported cases of suicide associated with it, as well as Parkinson-like symptoms such as shuffling gait, flat emotions and facial expressions, muscle tightness, and even drooling. The second-generation antipsychotics are notorious (although this is not communicated well enough, especially by pharmaceutical companies) for producing weight gain (not just a few pounds but tens of pounds), leading to insulin insensitivity and type 2 diabetes as well as disturbances in blood lipids, like cholesterol and triglycerides, which are harbingers of atherosclerosis in heart and brain arteries. All of the second-generation antipsychotic medications can sometimes cause significant sedation, apathy, loss of libido, and sometimes akathisia as well. Second, if a person has an illness that interferes with their capacity to appreciate that they are ill, why in the world would they take an unpleasant drug for an illness that others, like their parents, say they have, but they do not think they have. Finally, it is difficult to view medication as a blessing when an individual with a mental illness faces the prospect of contending with a lifetime of chronic illness. Putting a pill in your mouth can be a painful reminder of that reality.

The most controversial finding of CATIE was that no significant differences were found in how effective perphenazine was compared with the other four drugs in the first phase of the study. I recall when olanzapine and the other second-generation drugs received U.S. Food and Drug Administration approval and were marketed for the treatment of psychosis. They were heralded as "breakthrough" medications, welcomed by prescribing doctors like me for our patients, as well as by patients and their families, because they would not cause akathisia, drug-induced parkinsonism, and *tardive dyskinesia* (a late-onset movement disorder). Moreover, marketing for what was to become annual sales of billions of dollars for each new drug advertised that the second-generation agents would help with the negative symptoms of schizophrenia (like loss of motivation and apathy) as well as improve the cognitive deficits in executive mental functioning (like deterioration of attention, focus, memory, and task sequencing) that are so common when the disease becomes chronic. We would have more medication treatments—more would be better for sure. But more, CATIE revealed, was, in fact, not more in terms of treatment, and actually, often it was less.

An important measure of the utility and value of a medication (or any other treatment) is called *cost-effectiveness*. This means the clinical and social value that will derive from spending, say, a dollar on one treatment versus another. The escalating cost curves of medical care in this country scream out to legislators and citizens; we are spending nearly 20% of our gross national product on health care. That means there is less for education, roads, safety, housing, food, and other necessities. What's more, little of this huge health care budget is spent on prevention or early intervention—protecting the health of a population or mitigating early on the course of an illness. CATIE showed that an inordinate amount of money was being spent on second-generation medications that, overall, bestowed no greater therapeutic benefit on those who took the medications. Billions and billions of dollars, every year, funded the pharmaceutical companies, not community-based mental health services; CSC programs; and rehabilitation, skills-building, and recovery programs. More, a lot more, was being ill spent on second-generation, high-priced antipsychotic drugs when an equally effective, and far less costly, medication might do just as well.

There was one drug, clozapine, which proved itself more effective for those patients who did not respond to first-generation and other second-generation antipsychotics. Clozapine was approved for use in the United States in the late 1980s; it was expensive then and in short supply and raised many fears because of its rare but potential side effect of shutting down the bone marrow's production of white blood cells, thus rendering a person extremely vulnerable to infection and death. That was then. Now, its highly regulated dispensation, with registries and required blood monitoring of white cell counts, has made this danger to the patient's marrow virtually nonexistent; in fact, today more people die from clozapine-related bowel paralysis (also avoidable) than from an infection that is a consequence of a weakened immune system. Clozapine has been off patent for a long time and is inexpensive. This is an instance when more, a different type of medication, is actually more, rather than more of the same.

However, psychiatric practices have not followed the evidence that CATIE revealed. Second-generation antipsychotic drugs, the mainstay of expensive "me-too" products, continue to proliferate and cost as much as 100 times more than generic, first-generation and (now) second-generation generic drugs. Commentators about CATIE, as well as many families, remark about significant improvements or greater tolerability with newer medications and appropriately urge access lest a person with a serious mental illness be denied what may be working or might work. But psychiatric prescribing practices have not seen any increase in the prescription of first-generation drugs, whereas the ongoing love affair with what is new, marketed as different, and pricey remains unabated. The usage data for clozapine, a medication which has turned around the lives of many people with schizophrenia who did not respond to multiple trials of first- or second-generation antipsychotics, however, remain flat.

In my state government agency, we require our prescribers—more than 700 doctors and nurses who work for the 22 Office of Mental Health–operated hospitals and scores of outpatient clinics (where we often supply medication to uninsured patients)—to engage in a structured critical thinking exercise on antipsychotic medications (a type of checklist for themselves) and to make a case for using the newer, costly medications before they are dispensed (Sederer 2010). We operate on a fixed budget. If we spend millions on drugs that perform less well per dollar spent than comparable medications, then we have fewer dollars to spend on clinical staff and community services. Sometimes it is worth the extra money, but usually, it is not. Some managed-care companies administering mental health services require prior approval for a variety of medications. However, the experience of most prescribers is that "just say no" is often the ethos of these management companies; it generally is not a careful review of the cost benefit by senior medical staff, which is how we do it at my agency.

Our state mental health agency, as well, has made a concerted, multiyear effort to increase the use of clozapine, which is slowly work-

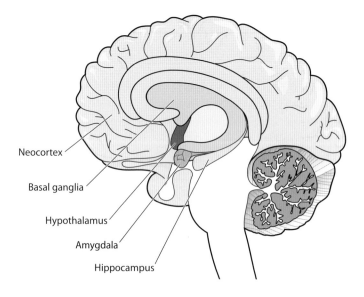

Neocortex

Basal ganglia

Hypothalamus

Amygdala

Hippocampus

Human hippocampus.

ing (Carruthers et al. 2016). About 18% of our patients, who are known to not have typically responded to multiple medication trials or who were on lots of different medications (polypharmacy, which is also not known to work for most patients) are taking clozapine, compared to a statewide average of less than 4% (national figures are also very low). Here again, we see that use of one comparably very affordable drug demonstrates how less money and fewer drugs can do more for patients and thus for their family and community.

In psychiatry, work is well underway to develop biomarkers (like DNA profiles or enzyme measures) that will better predict which patient will respond to which medication and at what point in their illness. When these biomarkers become part of our arsenal, we will be better able to see that less is more; we will not have to use a "shoot in the dark" methodology. But we are not there yet. Until then, doctors and nurses, administrators, policy gurus, patient and family advocates, and legislators need to support, at times insist on, practice patterns that are informed by evidence that acknowledges that antipsychotics, except for clozapine, manifest relatively equal effectiveness; they need to consider patient histories of response; and they need to examine and act upon cost-effectiveness data so that money can be repurposed to other than medication treatments. When that happens, we will have done more by doing less. That will not only help our patients and their families, it will honor a tradition of integrity in medical care that seems too often quashed by marketing and false promises. That is yet another secret worth spreading in mental health care.

False Memories

In a fascinating set of experiments, scientists at the Massachusetts Institute of Technology (MIT) were able to prove that mice could form false memories. *False memories*, convictions of individuals that something occurred that did not actually happen, have bedeviled mental health professionals faced with highly distressed people who assert they were sexually or physically abused in the past, as well as legal professionals faced with witnesses in courtrooms who provide testimony that could potentially convict someone of a heinous crime.

The MIT team focused on the hippocampus, the area of the brain, in mice and men, known to be associated with memory. Memory is established by a complex encoding process that includes both chemical and physical (connectivity) changes involving hippocampal brain cells. The scientists engineered changes in the brains of mice that would allow for a specific blue light to stimulate the hippocampus, thereby producing a protein involved in memory formation and recall. They then conditioned these mice to experience fear by placing them in a chamber, chamber A, where they would receive shocks to their feet. They then placed these mice in another chamber unlike the first, chamber B, where they were again given foot shocks while being exposed to the blue light, thereby conditioning a fear response (seen as freezing in mice) to this specific light color. Finally, the mice were placed in yet another chamber, C. When exposed to blue light in this setting, they demonstrated a fear response of the magnitude seen in chamber A even though they were not shocked in this new and different third setting. A false memory, stimulated by an association with a harmless light to electric shock, had been created in the mice, which had them respond fearfully to a situation that was not a danger to them. The control group did not show the same fearful response. These MIT scientists had shined a light, so to speak, on the neurobiological correlates of the phenomenon of false memory (Ramirez et al. 2013).

Cognitive studies have shown that humans, not just mice, show activity in the hippocampus during both genuine and false memories. Memory is dynamic and subject to many sources of input and alteration. What is going on demonstrates that our minds are not simply like cameras faithfully recording an event. Instead, our brains engage in a process of synthesizing (fabricating) memories from fragments of that event coupled with a myriad of internal associations, imaginings, experiences, and even dreams. This is not conscious or intentional, but it is universal. The result is great variability in the "truthfulness" of a memory: the result is the considerable unreliability of our memories.

When I was the chief medical officer at McLean Hospital outside of Boston, we had a specialty service for people, often women, with trauma disorders, usually not induced by disaster, war, torture, or forced relocation. Rather, they were suffering from dissociative disorders. They would arrive at the hospital by ambulance having done something painful to themselves, like severe cutting or burning or attempting suicide. Many had well-documented histories of physical or sexual abuse. Some of our patients told us that they were traumatized, although there was no medical or legal corroborating evidence, but that the trauma had been "retrieved" in the course of psychotherapy. For our short-term inpatient services, uncovering the cause of a person's traumatic or dissociative disorder was not the central concern at the time of the hospital stay (except of course if there was imminent external risk, such as domestic violence). Our work was to help the person find a place of psychological safety and calm, establish an effective community aftercare treatment plan, and foster hope for recovery. We rigorously avoided any exploration of past trauma or memories. Instead, our clinicians focused on the here and now and offered techniques and treatments for controlling and mastering intense feelings, fears, and self-destructive behaviors while they also mobilized family and community supports.

While this clinical care was taking place, other colleagues (in particular, Drs. Elizabeth Loftus and Paul McHugh) and other hospitals, such as McLean Hospital and Harvard University–affiliated hospitals, and university centers around the country were investigating what came to be known as false memory syndrome (FMS). FMS is a not uncommon condition in which a person believes with the same conviction as the mouse in chamber C that something happened to them in a particular setting or with a particular person that was egregiously painful and out of their control. The power of the memory disrupts the person's capacity to live effectively and renders them highly vulnerable to triggers. These triggers may be sensory experiences or incidents, what they feel in their bodies, see on TV, or hear from friends, which ignite a powerful, negative emotional response, which the affected person will do almost anything to avoid. Some individuals may even engage in various forms of self-injurious behavior to temper their psychic distress.

The consequences of false memory recovery do not stop with those experiencing the memories; they also extend to the loved ones and caregivers who are alleged to have perpetrated the abuse. Family members have been accused of abuse, and allegations have been promulgated against doctors and mental health professionals, which have led to court cases against therapists brought by patients claiming iatrogenic (doctor induced) harm. Some of these recovered memories include childhood abuse and even bizarre satanic rituals. Outside of my field, cases have occurred where false memories have prompted allegations of abuse in school and religious settings. Some consider UFO sightings and reports of alien abduction to stem from our ever-present capacity to create fiction from the world around us.

I do not mean to suggest that all recovered memories are false. Surely, some are indeed true. Did you see *Doubt*? What do you think happened in that fictitious story but very real play and movie?

False memory is especially catastrophic when the (false) memory is of a family member who is believed to have perpetrated the abuse.

Families can be shattered, and critical support for a person with genuine serious emotional problems is cut off by the false memory of abuse. The destructive force of false memory is very real. The life of the person who experiences these memories becomes profoundly compromised as they try to manage their distress either by avoidance or by devoting an inordinate amount of time, therapeutic attention, and resources in an attempt to extirpate them.

FMS achieved greater recognition because of clinical researchers investigating recovered memory therapy, a previously popular (and still persistent today) psychotherapy approach that seeks to uncover repressed memories and traumas considered by its proponents to be the genesis of a person's mental distress and disorganized life. Recovered memory therapy is entirely different from recognizing and acknowledging the tragedy and great prevalence of proven instances of childhood abuse, which is discussed in Chapter 4 ("Chronic Stress Is the Enemy") among other serious adverse childhood experiences. Adverse childhood experiences cry out not just for early detection and good treatment but also for far greater efforts at prevention. Recovered memory therapy, instead, actively pursues inquiry into a person's past using the influence of the therapist to suggest that a trauma did occur, when, in fact, it may not have. From what is known about FMS and human suggestibility, this is a type of therapy where more of that treatment is surely less of what the patient needs; a therapy that should be beneficial produces a worsening of symptoms and a life lived encumbered by a fiction generated by a bad, intensive psychotherapy. This seems all too reminiscent of pouring boiling oil on a wound that needs gentle healing.

The medical principle *primum non nocere* compels us. Less is (far) more when more is unnecessary. Less is (far) more when more gives rise to further psychopathology in people already suffering. People

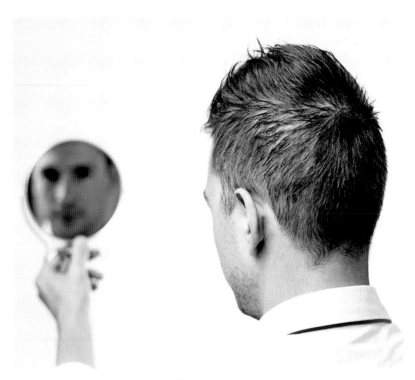

Examining ourselves.

with mental illness do not need to be further burdened by therapists who engender yet another layer of difficulty, an insoluble problem (because it is fabricated) that consequently leaves mice, men, and women with little to do but freeze in place.

———————————⬤———————————

It is difficult to write about this secret without appearing critical, with 20/20 hindsight about other people's excesses and mistakes. I hope that is not how this reads to you. That is not my intent. I, too, am only human and have made more than my fair share of mistakes.

However, it seems to me that to not declare **less as more** (in general) as one of the more common and consequential lessons in mental health care would be an irresponsible omission, and one meant to protect my profession from what is appropriate and necessary self-examination. The examples I have chosen are by no means comprehensive or necessarily what others might point to. But, they were chosen to illustrate how hard medical and mental health work can be and how sometimes the best of intentions, as has often been said, can pave the way to (therapeutic) hell. Or as my grandmother might have said (if this is not a false memory on my part), be careful because the less said and the less done may prove to be the more prudent of courses to take.

References

Carruthers J, Radigan M, Erlich MD, et al: An initiative to improve clozapine prescribing in New York state. Psychiatr Serv 67(4):369–371, 2016 26725299. Available at: http://ps.psychiatryonline.org/doi/full/10.1176/appi.ps.201500493.

Collins F: Study may RAISE standard for treating first psychotic episode. National Institutes of Health Director's blog, October 20, 2015. Available at: https://directorsblog.nih.gov/2015/10/20/study-may-raise-standard-for-treating-first-psychotic-episode/. December 28, 2015.

Drake RE, Sederer LI: The adverse effects of intensive treatment of chronic schizophrenia. Compr Psychiatry 27(4):313–326, 1986a 2873959

Drake RE, Sederer LI: Inpatient psychosocial treatment of chronic schizophrenia: negative effects and current guidelines. Hosp Community Psychiatry 37(9):897–901, 1986b 3758971

Lewis DA, Lieberman JA: Catching up on schizophrenia: natural history and neurobiology. Neuron 28(2):325–334, 2000 11144342

Lieberman JA, Stroup TS: The NIMH-CATIE Schizophrenia Study: what did we learn? Am J Psychiatry, 168(8): 770–775, 2011 21813492

Ramirez S, Liu X, Lin PA, et al: Creating a false memory in the hippocampus. Science 341(6144):387–391, 2013 23888038

Sederer LI: Is Your Doctor Using A Checklist? The Huffington Post, February 23, 2010. Available at: http://www.huffingtonpost.com/lloyd-i-sederer-md/is-your-doctor-using-a-ch_b_473068.html. Accessed December 28, 2015.

Swarz MS, Stroup TS, McEvoy JP, et al: What CATIE found: results from the schizophrenia trial. Psychiatr Serv 59(5):500–506, 2008 18451005

CHAPTER 4

CHRONIC STRESS IS THE ENEMY

The art of healing comes from nature, not from the physician. Therefore the physician must start from nature, with an open mind.

Paracelsus

The lion will lie down with the lamb, but the lamb won't get much sleep.

Woody Allen

When I met my new primary care doctor some years ago, she asked what my goals were. I said there were two: I wanted to minimize my body's chronic inflammatory processes and maximize my immune competency. I think she was bemused and asked me to say more, familiar as she was with these essential aspects of health.

I said that I understood that many physical disorders and aging processes in our bodies were the result of persistent inflammation in the blood vessels of the heart, brain, and other vital organs. I also thought that a variety of mental disorders, including depression, post-traumatic stress disorder (PTSD), and even schizophrenia, were linked to inflammation. I also knew that a state of persistent stress response can affect specific hormones that can compromise the body's capacity to defend against infection and detect and destroy abnormal cells, otherwise known as cancer. Persistent stress can also raise our blood pressure, putting strain on the heart and increasing the risk of heart attack and stroke.

Like most people, I want to live a long and healthy life. I just happen to also think about how we can achieve those ends, not just the ends in themselves. And so might you.

Adverse Childhood Experiences

For some people, exposure to sources (and consequences) of chronic stress begins at an early age.

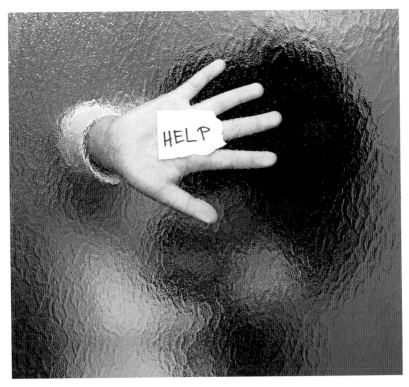

Child abuse.

Doreen Brant was born to a teenage mother who was herself physically abused and addicted to heroin. Doreen was placed in foster care at about 8 years old after she was sexually molested by her mother's boyfriend. By the time she was 14, she was obese, with prediabetes. She smoked cigarettes and was beginning to use synthetic marijuana (K2, Spice, etc.). She was frequently truant from school. Her foster parents, in her fifth home, reported that she was depressed and talked about taking her life.

Alberto Ruiz was 15 years old and had behavioral problems in school dating back almost a decade. His father was in prison for drug dealing. His mother had divorced his father, and her search for a stable male partner and father figure for her two sons yielded a series of unstable, volatile, and sometimes exploitative relationships. Alberto had multiple school suspensions and was at risk for expulsion because of fights and truancy. He started using tobacco, alcohol, and street drugs when he was 11.

The stories of these two teenagers are as tragic as they are common. These young people embody the consequences of adverse childhood experiences (ACEs), which can be seen in this or any other country. What these two youths share is that they both were exposed to a collection of ACEs. The initial study that identified the ACEs concept was done almost 20 years ago by the Centers for Disease Control and Prevention and the Kaiser Permanente Health Plan and involved over 17,000 participants (Felitti et al. 1998). The study explored childhood abuse and neglect and their aftermath. ACEs are events in the life of a child or adolescent that are beyond their control. These experiences can usher in a lifetime of misfortune and perpetuate a legacy of abuse and neglect in succeeding generations.

The principal types of ACEs are abuse, neglect, and seriously troubled households. More specifically, *ACEs are emotional, physical, and sexual abuse; emotional and physical neglect; and living in homes where there is domestic violence, mental and/or substance (alcohol or drug) disorders, parental separation or divorce, or a family member who is incarcerated.* ACEs are associated with risk for developing many of the following conditions and problems:

- Alcohol and drug abuse
- Depression
- Heart, lung, or liver disease
- Sexually transmitted diseases
- Intimate partner violence
- Smoking, including at an early age
- Suicide attempts
- Unintended pregnancies

As the number of ACEs that a youth experiences increase, so too does his or her risk for these problems and often before they depart their teen years! In fact, the greater the number of ACEs a youth experiences—and the presence of one ACE usually means there are others—the greater the likelihood of developing multiple physical, mental, and social problems. For example, children exposed to four or more categories of ACEs are at a fourfold to twelvefold increased risk of substance use problems, depression, and suicidal behavior. They are at a twofold to fourfold greater risk of smoking tobacco, poor (self-rated) health, having more than 50 sexual partners, and contracting sexually transmitted diseases. The risk of general medical disorders, such as cancer, ischemic heart disease, lung and liver diseases, and skeletal fractures, is also highly correlated with the increasing number of categories of ACEs to which an individual is exposed, with each additional ACE compounding future risk of disease, malaise, and a troubled life. ACEs are one of the most toxic forms of stress exposure that exists in our societies, and yet they seem to remain a secret in plain sight.

The principal means by which early-childhood adversity develops its toxic roots is thought to be the unregulated and ongoing release of stress hormones, including corticosteroids and adrenaline. These hormones weaken the body's defenses (compromising the immune system's ability to protect itself from infection and cancer), or, paradoxically, they activate our immune systems to turn against us (by destroying our own cells) in the form of autoimmune diseases like lupus, type 1 diabetes, multiple sclerosis, and rheumatoid arthritis. In addition, blood pressure is increased, plaque formation in arteries is promoted by the inflammatory process, and depressive and posttraumatic stress illnesses are fostered.

There are proven approaches to remedying the adversity of traumatic childhood, including the following:

- Home visits by nurses to mothers identified as being at high risk for emotional problems (e.g., Dr. David Olds' Nurse-Family Partnership Program)
- Primary care screening and early intervention for depression in moms
- Pediatric screening and early intervention for depression and addictive disorders in youth
- Parental skills training programs (e.g., ParentCorps, Positive Parenting, The Incredible Years, Bright Futures)
- Youth support programs (e.g., Big Brothers Big Sisters and many after-school programs)
- Pediatric medical homes that holistically support child development and deliver physical and mental health care and wellness services

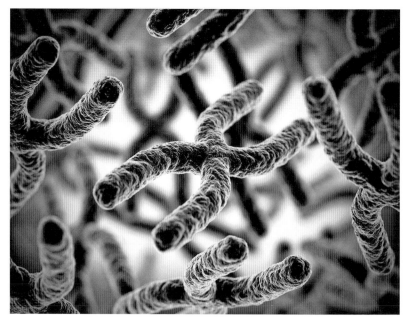

Telomeres.

- Trauma-focused mental health programs for youth already affected (e.g., Child and Family Traumatic Stress Intervention [Berkowitz et al. 2011])

Yet we have little evidence of efforts to widely disseminate these programs. The consequences are felt every day by our youths, families, communities, and pocketbooks.

Telomeres

Scientists at Stanford University, Northwestern University, and the University of California, San Francisco, recently reported on a study of 97 healthy girls, ages 10–14 (Gotlib et al. 2015). About half of the girls had moms with histories of depression, and about half had moms who did not. None of the girls had histories of depression. Saliva DNA samples were taken from all the girls.

Those girls whose moms had suffered depression had significant reductions in the length of their telomeres. We all want to understand *telomeres*, the caps at the ends of our DNA strands, because the longer they are, the longer we tend to live—and live freer of age-related illnesses like heart disease, stroke, dementia, diabetes, and osteoporosis. A long and healthy life, as our toasts proclaim for us, is in part dictated by our telomeres. The girls whose moms didn't have histories of depression, the control group of the study, did not show the same changes in their DNA as a result of reductions (wearing away) in the length of their telomeres.

The researchers took the study a step further: they compared both groups of girls, the former or high-risk group and the control or low-risk group, by measuring their responses to stressful mental tasks. The children of moms with depression had significantly higher levels of cortisol, a principal corticosteroid stress hormone, released during these tasks than those in the control group; both had normal levels of cortisol before the stressful tasks.

These findings are what scientists call *associations*, namely, highly significant events found together that are unlikely to co-occur randomly. In themselves, they don't prove one caused the other, but they suggest (with degrees of certainty) that something important, not accidental, is going on. What this study demonstrated was that daughters of moms who had depression had shorter telomeres and greater hormonal reactivity to stress.

The girls were then followed until age 18. Sixty percent of those in the high-risk group developed depression, a condition that was not present when they were first studied. In other words, we might consider telomere length to be a *biomarker*, a hallmark that indicates some phenomenon—in this case, the risk for depression. We already knew that shortened telomeres were a risk factor for chronic, physical diseases, but now evidence is emerging for their likely role in depression.

Should you go out and get your saliva tested? I imagine there are labs that would be happy to provide the test. But your decision should depend on whether you have reason to suspect being at risk, like a family history of maternal depression, which may be all you actually need to know. Keep in mind that information is most valuable when we can do something about it.

And we can. We have a growing set of tools to help control our stress responses, including yoga, yogic breathing, meditation, cognitive-behavioral therapy, exercise, diet, and ongoing efforts to have supportive, stable relationships in home and work environments. People at greater risk for stress-related diseases (mind you, we all are at risk it's just a matter of degree) would be wise to learn and master these techniques early in life and to use them to live a healthier and longer life. Is this prescription routinely offered by mental health and addiction professionals and programs that serve people with and at risk for depression and other mental health conditions? Not exactly.

As clinicians, we also need to better detect and treat mothers who suffer from depression. We have strong evidence that untreated depression in new moms impairs their attachment to their children and is associated with these children developing behavioral and emotional problems in childhood. If the moms are properly treated, not only do they fare better, so do their kids.

Understanding genetic predispositions, developing reliable biomarkers, teaching patients to manage their environments and stresses to protect themselves from harmful hormones, and promoting access to effective treatments for the disorders that do arise may be the best prescription for healthier and longer lives—and not a secret to keep to ourselves.

Social Determinants of Mental Health

With all the attention, at least in the United States, to advancing innovation in medical care, we seldom stop to consider that *medical treatments* account for a mere 10% of what constitutes our physical and mental health. Ninety percent of the determinants of our health, in fact, derive from our lifetime social and physical environments. Americans are prone to confound health care with health.

What does account for our health (both physical and mental) is related principally to how and where we live our lives (Centers for Disease Control and Prevention 2014). Poor eating (too much and foods that over the course of time overwhelm our pancreas and invite clogging of our arteries); excessive drinking and drug use; smoking; physical inactivity; and high intake of salt are huge drivers of ill health and abbreviated life spans. They are the culprits responsible for the lion's share (40%) of our ill health and early demise (Compton and Shim 2015; Sederer 2016).

Lower income (poverty) and lower social status are also linked to poorer health, and their inverses are associated with better health. The greater the income gap between groups, the greater their health disparities. Lower education levels are also associated with poorer health and greater stress. Safe water and clean air and reliable and safe housing also contribute to well-being. Employed people are healthier than those who are unemployed. And supportive families and friends are connected to better health.

In short, it is our lifestyle and our environment that account for 40% of our physical and mental health problems and premature death. In addition, while an estimated 30% of our health is attributable to our genes, we now also understand (through the science of epigenetics) that genes are turned on or off by their exposure to our environment and how we lead our lives, thereby adding more factors, other than health care, as determinants of health. In other words, behaviors and environment are the dominant factors that determine longevity and quality of life. They are, therefore, what we will need to grapple with to make a real difference in our health and that of our families and communities.

It is very likely, at least in part, that the adversities of our social circumstances and our less than healthy behaviors do their ongoing damage by stoking our immune system and mobilizing a chronic inflammatory response in our bodies. The misfortunes of birth and/or environment and our own harmful behaviors that we perpetrate and the chronic stresses they evoke are the principal foes of physical and mental well-being and the achievement of a long life, well lived.

Mind you, if you or I (or my loved ones) get sick, I am all for the most effective, affordable, and accessible medical, mental health, and addiction treatments. Indeed, I have spent my career trying to deliver such treatment. I want to go to the best doctor, clinic, or hospital. I want to take treatments that work and don't break my bank account or cause intolerable side effects. I am just saying that's what we need if and when we get sick, not what we need to avert or limit sickness in the first place.

Scientists have long explored how our bodies evolved to produce the *stress response*—the automatic, immediate mobilization of our minds and bodies that enables vulnerable humans (and other higher-order organisms) to survive. What seems well understood, at least until it is replaced by a greater understanding of the brain, hormones, and bodily organs, is that a stressor—like the scent or sight of a predator or a dangerous object rapidly advancing toward us and about to do grave harm—is first recognized in the brain. A message (a neat term meant to summarize and explain how in the world a smell or sight is perceived, recognized, decoded, and understood as dangerous) is relayed to the hypothalamus, a small area deep in the evolutionarily ancient brain, which discharges corticotropin-releasing hormone (see the illustration of the hypothalamic-pituitary-adrenal axis) into the pituitary gland. A cascade of more noticeable events ensues. This takes seconds at most.

The pituitary releases into the bloodstream adrenocorticotropic hormone (ACTH), also called corticotropin because of its tropic (growth) or production-inducing effect on corticosteroids, the most familiar being cortisol. ACTH is like a hormonal bullet that rapidly finds its way to our adrenal glands, which sit firmly atop our kidneys. The adrenals respond by releasing epinephrine (also known as adrenaline) and norepinephrine (noradrenaline) with amazing speed; this produces the famous fight-or-flight response with its increased heart and respiration rates, constriction of arteries meant to limit bleeding but

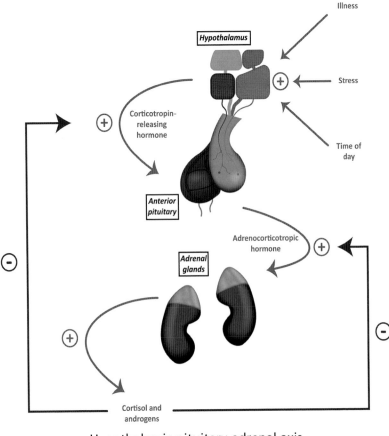

Hypothalamic-pituitary-adrenal axis.

also raising blood pressure, deviation of blood flow away from the gut and into the muscles, and a state of alarmed wakefulness. Some say that this response is more pronounced in men, perhaps mitigated in women by the release of oxytocin, the bonding or affiliative hormone, but that is another matter beyond this all too short explanation.

The adrenaline burst is like a sprint: it is meant to be brief and intense. What keeps the response going is the adrenal release of corticosteroids, which can sustain the stress response for minutes, hours, or even longer. When the corticosteroid release does not subside as it should when the danger is past, we enter a state of chronic stress and with that chronic inflammation and immune dysfunction can develop.

Let's look a bit further at the inflammatory response. An acute inflammatory response is what happens when we cut our skin or have a serious bout of hay fever or poison ivy. The affected site, like our wounded or irritated skin or allergic nasal passages, gets red, swollen, hot, and painful. That's the inflammatory response at work as certain types of our white blood cells release specific chemicals that open nearby blood vessels and release fluid, histamine, and other substances to produce the reaction. Acute inflammation is good—it prevents infection and promotes tissue healing.

But when acute inflammation becomes chronic (because the stress response has not appropriately subsided) and, for example, goes after healthy tissue, that's not good at all. That's what happens in atherosclerotic vessels in the heart and brain, causing heart attacks and strokes. That's what appears to be part of the disease process in the brains of people with Alzheimer's disease, in the joints of those with rheumatoid arthritis, and in the pancreases of those with diabetes. It is also likely going on in a variety of cancers. For the tens of millions of Americans taking statins such as Lipitor and Crestor because their

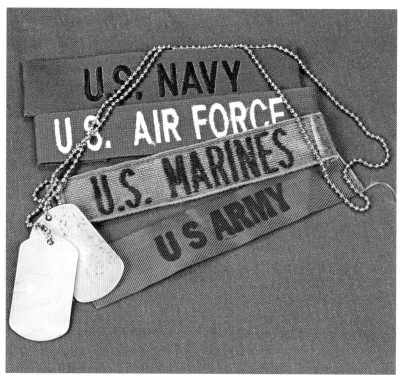
U.S. military tags.

low-density lipoproteins (LDLs or "lousy" lipids) are too high, the most likely benefit is reduction of the inflammation in their cardiac arteries, which prevents further buildup of fatty deposits and other unwelcome junk, which is drawn to the inflamed walls and produces highly undesirable plaques that restrict the passage of blood.

When scientists pursue the holy grail of what causes aging (and therefore what might prevent senescence and keep us forever young), modesty on the part of the smartest of the lot has them tell us that why we age still remains a mystery. But one of their prime suspects is chronic inflammation.

Posttraumatic Stress Disorder

John Orlando had returned from his third tour in Afghanistan when I met him. A decorated soldier, now in the reserves, he had seen combat, lost men with whom he served and whom he commanded, and witnessed the extremes of the brutality of war. He was in treatment for combat-related PTSD. While he was laconic in describing his problems, his wife, Debbie Orlando, spoke for him: he woke every night with nightmares that either repeated his war experiences or were dream-like versions of them; most every night he drank a six-pack or more of beer (even though he was taking antidepressant medication) to relax and to try to enable sleep to come. He seemed "out of touch" with his family, including his two children, because he had retreated into himself, yet loud noises, sudden movements, or situations that reminded him of his time at war evoked in him intense fear and a readiness to strike out aggressively. At times, Mrs. Orlando feared for herself and her children because of how out of control her husband could become at a moment's unexpected provocation. She insisted that all weapons be removed from their home and kept safely locked up with Mr. Orlando's brother.

PTSD derives from having experiences where a person's life or physical safety is endangered, or it feels as if it is, or a person witnesses the serious threat or actual harm to others. While it is well known that war can cause PTSD (over the ages it has had a variety of names), it is a condition that can occur in the wake of disaster, torture, and forced dislocation from home or country and from physical, sexual, and emotional abuse. Its hallmark symptoms, such as Mr. Orlando experienced, are nightmares, flashbacks to the traumatic event(s), intrusive thoughts and images, startle reactions, and avoidance of any triggers (e.g., feelings, memories, circumstances) that can stimulate a fear response.

What causes PTSD remains a highly active area of scientific inquiry. There appear to be genetic, epigenetic (where genes are turned on or off by the vagaries of our lives), and a variety of abnormal hormonal, neurochemical, and other biological processes in our brains and bodies that are associated with the disorder. A growing body of evidence now points to the role of (chronic) inflammation in the genesis and maintenance of PTSD, a condition all too common in the members of our military.

An elegant set of studies performed by researchers at New York University, the University of California, San Francisco, and Stanford University reveals that chronic inflammation appears to be significantly involved in combat-related PTSD (Lindqvist et al. 2014). What was discovered was that PTSD is independent of depression and early-life stress. Combat-exposed veterans (all men in this study) with and without PTSD (reliably diagnosed) had their blood sampled for the presence of a group of inflammatory markers (e.g., interleukin, interferon, tumor necrosis factor, and C-reactive protein); the results on these markers were combined to create a "proinflammatory" score, a composite index of the degree to which their bodies were besieged by inflammation. The soldiers with PTSD had significantly higher scores than those who did not have this condition; careful attention was paid to ensure that the results were not confounded by the presence of other conditions (e.g., asthma or allergies, depression, physical illnesses), taking medications, or experiencing trauma earlier in their lives. The more severe a soldier's PTSD, the higher, on average, was his proinflammatory score.

An extensive analysis (some 300 studies) also has demonstrated that chronic psychological stress is disruptive to our immune system (Lohr et al. 2015). For example, natural killer (NK) cells are part of the human immune response system; NK cells are exceptionally attuned to protect us from viruses and tumors (even better than their more well-known cousins the T cells). These first-line defenders of our health, well-being, and longevity show significantly impaired protective capabilities in people with histories of chronic stress.

Related work by some of the same New York University scientists and their colleagues (who express regret about how limited research with women has been to date) who reported on the combat veterans also looked at their NK cells. By comparing combat-exposed men with and without PTSD, they showed that those with PTSD had significant disturbances in the functioning of their NK cells, whereas those without PTSD did not. Chronic stress was destroying the ability of these men to defend against infectious disease and cancer, an awful price for them to pay for their service. There is even evidence that markers of aging (like shortened telomeres, intracellular mitochondrial DNA mutations, and increased proinflammatory markers as discussed earlier) are more pronounced in people with PTSD, cutting lives short in addition to inducing suffering along the way (Lindqvist et al. 2014).

It is not (yet) known whether the inflammatory state discovered in these men results from exposure to emotional and physical stress or if the inflammatory agents released in our bodies may themselves produce the symptoms of PTSD. But PTSD (and other conditions, but let's stick with this condition for the moment) has long been proven to be associated with states (in animals) where there are disturbances in the sympathetic nervous system (the fight-or-flight response with norepinephrine as its agent) and in the hypothalamic-pituitary-adrenal (HPA) axis (malfunction with corticosteroids and corticotropin-releasing hormone as its agents, see illustration).

Norepinephrine increases our heart and respiration rate as well as our blood pressure. It sends a danger message to the body to ready us for a struggle for survival. We wouldn't do very well in acutely dangerous situations without it. Norepinephrine also activates a region in our brains (actually two little almond shaped bodies of cells, one on each side of the brain) called the amygdala, intensifying our capacity to remember the source of danger, conditioning us to a specific fear, like the approach of an aggressive animal or oncoming bus, and thereby increasing the likelihood of survival over time. This helps to explain why people with PTSD avoid triggers, which have been encoded into memory as if they are true threats to life and limb. It turns out, conversely, that resilience to life-threatening stress (the capacity to tolerate extreme stress and not get sick) appears to be linked to a decreased responsiveness of the amygdala.

Corticosteroids are the other friend or foe, depending on whether they quiet down when their work is done. Cortisol is a corticosteroid that stimulates the adrenals and the body's inflammatory response (recall that we need that response to fight infection and promote wound healing). However, when the HPA system (a type of balanced loop that tries to both respond with a burst of activity and then return to normal levels) is disrupted, the inflammatory response just keeps on going; it keeps on chronically firing away and causing imbalance and disease in a host of organs susceptible to its effects. Chronic release of corticosteroids as well as aberrations in their feedback loops suppresses the immune system, leaving us at greater risk for infection and tumor growth.

Too little work has been done examining inflammation in women veterans and in children. But what research we have, especially in youths, seems to tell the same story of how unmitigated and unrelenting (chronic) stress is the enemy (Weissman et al. 2006).

I recall asking one seasoned soldier who had been exposed to firefights, improvised explosive devices, and combat death why he thought he could sleep well at night and did not suffer from PTSD like many in his squad. He said, "I must be wired differently." I guess he must have been referring to his HPA system, his amygdala, and the range of body functions and organs they impact.

Depression

Depression is the poster child of psychiatric disorders: It is highly prevalent (in all countries), commonly travels as a copilot with a host of other medical diseases (such as diabetes, heart disease, stroke, Parkinson's disease, cancer, asthma, and other chronic illnesses), is understood by the general public, and can be effectively treated. I am referring to clinical depression, major depressive disorder—not passing blue moods or a bad hair day—where darkness of mood prevails for weeks, months, or years.

For depression, the "central mood," noted by Emily Dickinson, is bleak, hopeless, and absent of life's everyday pleasures. Untreated, as it very often is, depression can be debilitating. It is the "black dog" that steals a person's energy, motivation, concentration, affection, hope, and will to live. Each year in the United States, over 42,000 people take their lives by suicide, and the vast preponderance of them are clinically depressed.

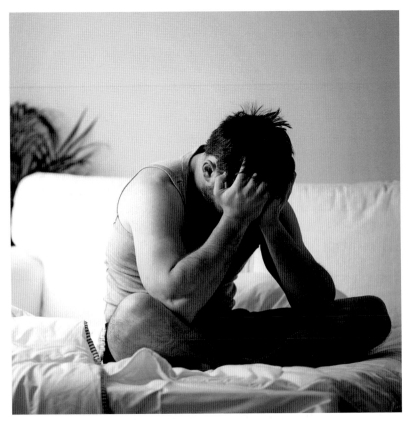

Depression.

Depression is another illness where chronic inflammation, mobilized by chronic stress, manifests its toxic effects and does its damage. People with major (clinical) depression show elevated levels of the biomarkers of inflammation, such as C-reactive protein. Our knowledge of how sustained, chronic stress may lead to depression remains rudimentary. Perhaps it is by adversely affecting the way brain circuits operate, whether they harmonize or fail to with each other? Perhaps it is by wreaking havoc with brain neurotransmitters like serotonin, dopamine, epinephrine, or glutamate? Perhaps it is through an infection (maybe in utero) that stimulates an immune reaction, with its inflammatory response? These same considerations apply to schizophrenia and bipolar disorders. Perhaps it is by impeding *neurogenesis* (the development of nervous system tissue), a more contemporary view of one possible aspect of the underlying pathology of depression? And perhaps no single explanation could possibly fit every depressed person.

Brain imaging studies have shown reduced size (indicating cell loss) of the hippocampus, a critical brain structure located below the cortex and instrumental to memory, in many people with depression. There are hypotheses that antidepressants like Prozac, Paxil, and Effexor work not so much by increasing brain neurotransmitters (the theory that has prevailed for a while) but by restoring the brain's capacity for neurogenesis, including in the hippocampus. The use of anti-inflammatory agents has been proposed as a treatment for depression. Unfortunately, there is little evidence that such agents like aspirin or ibuprofen, at least alone, are effective antidepressants, but they may augment the efficacy of antidepressants in some people.

I would be remiss if I did not mention at least two other ubiquitous disorders that afflict countless people globally: anxiety and substance use disorders. Anxiety disorders are like the fight-or-flight response on (anabolic) steroids, if you will pardon the (other) steroid analogy.

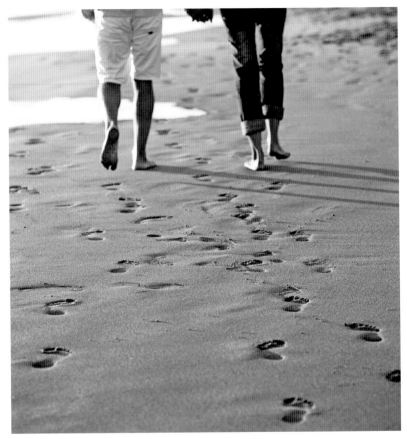

Make the path by walking it.

With addiction, which is a whole field unto itself, reward (pleasure) pathways are hijacked by alcohol and other drugs, as expressed by the proverb, "Man takes a drink, drink takes a drink, drink takes the man." For people with serious anxiety and substance use disorders, stress is surely part of what aggravates their conditions. And given how little we know about the underlying mechanisms of these common, often co-occurring conditions, chronic stress should be considered, as they say in police terminology, a "person of interest" if not an actual suspect.

So much unhappiness, so much distress, so much dysfunction, so much more to learn.

What We Can Do

Our understanding of how chronic stress produces or worsens so many ailments remains limited and often speculative. We see the association of stress with the body's inflammatory responses, with the HPA axis, with the hippocampus and amygdala, with impaired immune functioning, and with neurotransmitters and neurogenesis; but this is only what the investigative tools we have today permit us to appreciate. Scientists 100 years from now will probably chuckle about how simplistic or downright wrong the theories of their early twenty-first-century counterparts were in explaining the pathogenesis and pathophysiology of chronic diseases and their links to chronic stress.

But our limited knowledge of why need not keep us from taking a variety of actions to prevent stress and to mitigate its harm.

The greatest preventive actions to improve the physical and mental health of the inhabitants of this earth are the most universal—and challenging. These are the actions focused on the social determinants of physical and mental health discussed earlier in this chapter (Compton and Shim 2015). This means guaranteeing the availability of safe housing; relief from food insecurity and provision of nutritious diets; freedom from corrosive poverty; protection from domestic and community violence; accessibility of comprehensive prekindergarten through high school education; the opportunity for employment and a living wage; and the obliteration of class and ethnic stigma, discrimination, and injustice. Improvements made in each one of these determinants not only will make for a healthier global population, it will raise the collective morality of humankind. These are goals that are as hard to achieve as they are critical. But because it is a matter of collective human will, perseverance, and a bit of good fortune, we might actually succeed.

For individuals, folks like you and me, are there actions we can take today—or maybe plan for tomorrow? Ask any good (informed) doctor what the one most effective thing is that you can do to improve your health and live longer, and you should hear "exercise." You don't have to go at it like Arnold Schwarzenegger or be Mr. (or Ms.) Universe. Walking regularly, 10,000–12,000 steps a day, will help a lot. Try to get some good sleep because sleep deprivation in youths and adults mobilizes our stress response and dulls our minds and judgments. Naps can help too; Charlie Rose is big on naps, so was Oliver Sacks, and I am too.

You can go vegan or paleo or maybe just try a Mediterranean diet, but stay away from processed foods, refined sugar, too much salt, saturated fats, and lots of red meat and French fries. Don't eat too much. Drink alcohol in moderation. Don't smoke or use other forms of tobacco. Stay away from street drugs, which are loaded with lovely things like rat poison and chemicals manufactured in China and Russia that can induce psychosis or simply stop you from breathing.

Even Marines and corporate executives are learning to meditate to lower their heart rate and blood pressure as well as to improve their focus, productivity, and creativity. I like yogic breathing, slow breathing of six breaths a minute with slight resistance on exhalation, which can be done anywhere, anytime, even while waiting at a red light or in a boring meeting.

Positive thinking is good protection against stress and beneficial to our health. The American philosopher and psychologist William James, perhaps presaging today's cognitive-behavioral treatments, said, "The greatest weapon against stress is our ability to choose one thought over another." That can take some training and practice, like slow breathing or meditation, but it is not just for the rich and famous.

Faith, too, helps with health, well-being, and resilience to stress. Not everyone, far fewer people today than ever, engages in a religion which supports belief in a higher being or entity. But faith need not be only religious in nature, dependent on an institutionalized system of belief, a deity, and specific practices. Faith can also take the form of spirituality, a view that a higher power exists, that the universe is not chaos, that purpose in life is possible and essential, and that God is immanent, all around and in us.

Last but certainly not least, in our personal campaigns for well-being is the caring and support of others. They can be family, friends, lovers, comrades in arms, or fellow pilgrims on the adventure trail of life. As the proverb says, "If you want to go fast, go alone. If you want to go far, go with others."

References

Berkowitz SJ, Sover CS, Marans SR: The Child and Family Traumatic Stress Intervention: secondary prevention for youth at risk of developing PTSD. J Child Psychol Psychiatry 52(6):676–685, 2011 20868370

Centers for Disease Control and Prevention: NCHHSTP Social Determinants of Health: definitions. March 21, 2014. Available at http://www.cdc.gov/

nchhstp/socialdeterminants/definitions.html. Accessed December 28, 2015.

Compton MT, Shim RS: The Social Determinants of Mental Health. Arlington, VA, American Psychiatric Publishing, 2015

Felitti VJ, Anda RF, Nordenberg D, et al: Relationship of childhood abuse and household dysfunction to many of the leading causes of death in adults: The Adverse Childhood Experiences (ACE) Study. Am J Prev Med 14(4):245–258, 1998 9635069

Gotlib IH, LeMoult J, Colich NL, et al: Telomere length and cortisol reactivity in children of depressed mothers. Mol Psychiatry 20(5):615–620, 2015 25266121

Lindqvist D, Wolkowitz OM, Mellon S, et al: Proinflammatory milieu in combat-related PTSD is independent of depression and early life stress. Brain Behav Immun 42:81–88, 2014 24929195

Lohr JB, Palmer BW, Eidt CA, et al: Is post-traumatic stress disorder associated with premature senescence? A review of the literature. Am J Geriatr Psychiatry 23(7):709–725, 2015 25959921

Sederer LI: The social determinants of mental health. Psychiatr Serv 67(2):234–235, 2016, 26522677

Weissman MM, Pilowsky DJ, Wickramaratne PJ, et al: Remissions in maternal depression and child psychopathology: a STAR*D-child report. JAMA 295(12):1389–1398 2006 16551710

SOME CONCLUDING THOUGHTS

We cannot direct the wind,
but we can adjust our sails.

Henry David Thoreau

Perhaps, we mental health practitioners as well as our patients and their families (because we are all in this together) have developed some bad habits, ones so automatic that they escape our notice and prevent our seeing what is in plain sight.

The French philosopher Michel de Montaigne wrote in his essay on custom:

> For in truth habit is a violent and treacherous schoolmistress. She establishes in us, little by little, stealthily, the foothold of her authority; but having by this mild and humble beginning settled and planted it with the help of time, she soon uncovers to us a furious and tyrannical face against which we no longer have the liberty of even raising our eyes.

Failing to understand that a behavior is serving a purpose seems a habit worth changing because it has the power to distance us from those we serve and care about. Not appreciating that a human touch, a connection made, an attachment fostered, which are the greatest anodynes against isolation and despair, seems a sad habit that deprives us all—caregivers and recipients alike. Doing more may appear to be a virtue, but it is not when good intentions are thwarted or another layer of malaise results. Finally, preserving habits that may have been spawned by adversity but no longer serve our patients is incompatible with healing. Our lives are upended not by the stress of predators and acute dangers but by psychic trauma, environmental toxins, social misfortune, and lifestyles of abundance that our bodies, limited by the pace of our evolution, can hardly tolerate. These struggles demand new ways of responding.

Montaigne not only shines a light on the forces of habit, he also wisely suggests that a habit's origin is often humble and thus may elude notice. I would add that a behavior may have arisen and become a habit because it was helpful to an individual or a species; it is only when the habit takes on a life of its own *and* endures even when it is no longer productive that we have a problem. What should be plainly obvious can be obscured by patterns of thought and behavior that are no longer constructive.

What makes habits all the more devilish is that they are really hard to change. Such is the nature of habit, and such is the human condition. First, habitual behaviors can evade our awareness. We often don't even know we are jumping to conclusions or turning away from a source of sustenance or support. Second, we may have certain reasons, like the limited value we still obtain from doing something in a known and familiar way or because we fear doing something different, for not wanting to change a habit even when, in fact, we are aware of it. Third, habits go about their business in rather automatic ways that typically bypass our conscious attention, which is generally focused elsewhere (think about how you can drive home without considering each twist and turn and still arrive at your final destination). A habit originally adopted to solve a problem can outlive its effectiveness and become simply self-perpetuating.

I know about habits that erode our hopes and the quality of our existence because I have succumbed to them and labored to escape them as well. I also have spent a career trying to help people make better lives for themselves, their families, and their communities by understanding what they want and then acting in ways that optimize the likelihood of achieving those aims, be they relationships, purpose, self-esteem, productivity, or dignity. In offering this book, I do so with the humility of a fellow frail human being and with the belief that we all can change, solve problems, and make better lives for ourselves and those we love and value.

The secrets discussed in each chapter of this book—purposeful behavior, attachment, less can (often) be more, and the enemy of chronic stress—are each accompanied by some strategies to try to pry no longer useful habits loose and send them on their way. However, what remedies I offer are cursory: this is less a book about therapeutics and behavior change than it is an exploration of some of the dark avenues of our lives that need more streetlights and pedestrian traffic. When streets are well lit and well travelled, they become zones of safety and prosperity. Ask any urbanist, not just me.

We humans occupy a position of dominance in our environment because we have developed extraordinary cerebral cortices. We are blessed with resilience, the capacity to rebound after adversity, to rebuild neighborhoods and neurons. Our experiences, which are enriched by friends, family, and community, allow us to renew and regenerate. Those billions of cortical cells and their vast dendritic connections, however, are of limited power when it comes to changing habits. Habit is automatic and an awesome foe to even the most determined because it can operate independently of cortical control. Try resisting pizza, chips, peanut M&Ms, or a drink when you are tired, stressed, or lonely. Try resisting an addiction or an obsessional ritual by will alone. We need to channel the relentless tide of habit, until we have redirected its currents to power more beneficial behaviors.

Acting on the truths within these secrets and altering habits gone awry are both individual and societal endeavors.

For individuals, especially those seeking mental health care, we need to invest more in prevention and early intervention. Efforts at prevention have generally met with limited success because of how little we know (so far) about preventing mental and addictive disorders. We have not put enough emphasis on early intervention for psychosis, depression, posttraumatic stress disorder, addiction, and other common mental conditions because that would require upsetting a medical and mental health system that has specialized in taking care of sick people, not keeping people from getting sick.

Our experience in New York State has shown us how difficult it is to screen and treat depression in the primary care setting and to introduce statewide innovative and effective early-treatment programs for youths with psychosis. We are getting there, but not fast enough for those people who need better services *today*. Psychiatric treatments for those who have become acutely or chronically ill are fairly good; their efficacy is comparable to treatments for general medical conditions. But there is so much more to be done—discoveries of new technologies that alter brain circuits and hormonal regulatory mechanisms and the advancement of personalized medicine that allows us to better identify which treatment will work for which patient at what phase of an illness.

But recall, as I wrote earlier, only 10% (!) of our health is determined by health care. Health care alone is a thin reed in the storm of illness and despair that afflicts our species. I want it when I need it, but I really don't want to need it. Greater solutions lie in the social determinants of physical and mental health. This is an arena beyond the psychiatrist's or mental health practitioner's office, but it is one where we need to make our voices heard and to engage our efforts. The effects of trauma and stigma are clearly in our wheelhouse; but violence, housing and food instability, inadequate wages, social discrimination, and lack of educational opportunity are everyone's business, including the helping professions. I am not talking about mental health solutions (alone) to remedy universal social problems, but I am talking about mental health professionals joining teams to help create the (social) policies, practices, and conditions that can alter the destructive tides eroding our lives day after day, year after year.

I love my field, my work, and the good my profession can do. I wish we could do more, which is why I wrote this book. I want to offer what I can here, by presenting a few words that might enable healers practicing today to do more by seeing what might be right before their eyes, even if seeing is difficult and changing is even harder. I want all of us who have the privilege of teaching and guiding to provide the next generation of professionals with more tools and wisdom than we received. And, with both modesty and hope, I want all of us to usher in a better society for the generations who will follow in our footsteps.

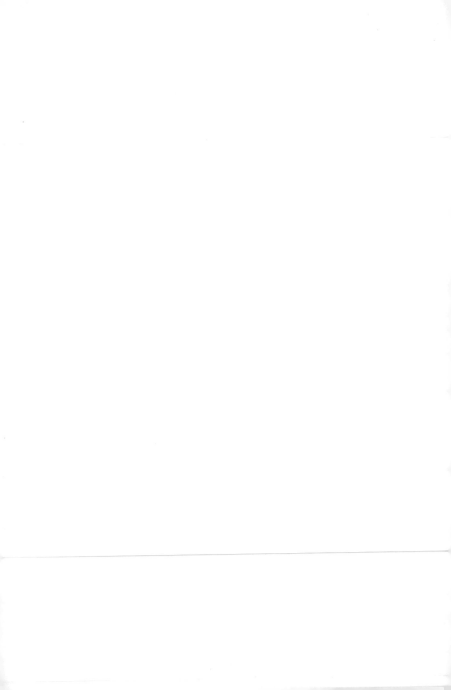